A Teen
Eating Disorder
Prevention
Book

Understanding
Exercise
Addiction

Marlys Johnson

The Rosen Publishing Group, Inc./New York

Published in 2000 by The Rosen Publishing Group, Inc.
29 East 21st Street, New York, NY 10010

First Edition

Library of Congress Cataloging-in-Publication Data

Johnson, Marlys.
   Understanding exercise addiction / Marlys Johnson.
      p. cm. (A teen eating disorder awareness book)
   Includes bibliographical references and index.
   Summary: Discusses addiction to exercise, its relationship to diet diseases like bulimia and anorexia, its causes, and what can be done to overcome it.
   ISBN 0-8239-2990-6 (lib. bdg.)
   1. Exercise addiction—Juvenile literature. [1. Exercise addiction. 2. Eating disorders.] I. Title. II. Series.
   RC569.5E94 J64 2000
   616.86—dc21   99-042550
                                     CIP
                                     AC

Manufactured in the United States of America

ABOUT THE AUTHOR

Marlys Johnson, M.Ed., LPC, worked as a children's and family therapist for seven years. For four years, she worked directly with the chemically dependent. She was a children's therapist at a women's residential treatment program, McCambridge Center in Columbia, Missouri. She has also worked as a teacher and behavioral consultant. Currently, Ms. Johnson is a journalist and freelance writer. She has written more than fifty articles on various topics, including health and business, and profiles of people of interest.

Contents

Introduction

Remember how you started exercising? You and your girlfriends hit the running track after seeing how good Britney Spears looked in her new music video. Or you wanted to be like Tiger Woods, a professional athlete at the top of his golf game, and you started to work on your golf swing. Soon you were working out regularly. Once you got into it, you liked the way it made you feel, how buffed and toned you looked, how pumped up you were, ready to try new things, maybe even ask the girl next to you in math class for a date. But something has changed.

Now you run and work out because you feel you have no choice. You schedule your day around it. You reschedule other activities and put things off so that you have time to exercise. You put off family, homework, and boyfriends or girlfriends because of your need to work out. You may even skip school or quit a job so that you can exercise. You exercise in spite of illness, injury, or threatening conditions like thunderstorms and icy roads. You exercise against the advice of your physician after you get an injury. If you do not work out, you feel anxious, depressed, restless, or you can't sleep at night. Sound like an addiction? It is.

Exercise addiction, like other addictions, takes over your life. It changes from something you do to keep fit and healthy to something that you have to do even if your health suffers because of it. Addiction changes something as healthy as exercise into something negative, something harmful. Overexercising causes injuries, exhaustion, degeneration of muscles and joints, back problems, and more. It causes problems with your family relationships, your schoolwork, and your social life. No matter what the consequences, when you are addicted to exercise you cannot stop working out. The urge to exercise is too strong. Exercise is your solution to everything. If you had a bad day, you go to an aerobics class to make yourself feel better. If you do not have a date for the weekend, you lift weights instead.

Teens exercise for different reasons. Many teens exercise as a way to control their weight, to purge themselves of calories. They reason that it doesn't matter if they had a double burger with fries for lunch; they will burn it off later when they work out. You can have butter on your popcorn at the movies if you want to, and maybe even a package of chocolate mints, because you will go to the gym later and work it off. Many times the compulsion to exercise is part of an eating disorder. An estimated 4 to 5 percent of all teenagers and young adult females have either bulimia or anorexia, two common eating disorders involving self-starvation. Young males are reporting problems with eating disorders more than ever before.

Teens become addicted to exercise in many different sports. Running, cycling, and aerobics are the most common sports where exercise addictions occur. But you can become addicted to swimming, tennis, golf, basketball, skateboarding, weight lifting, and almost any other sports activity. You can become addicted to exercise or a sports activity either physically or psychologically.

Teens want to be able to exercise and to look fit and healthy. Treating an exercise addiction is about learning to enjoy exercising again, to manage your exercise workouts so that the need to exercise does not manage you. Changing the goals of your exercise workout is a good place to start. When you shift the focus of your workout away from trying to sculpt the perfect body—something that is impossible to achieve—to having a healthy one, you will be exercising for the right reasons again, and you will feel a lot better about yourself.

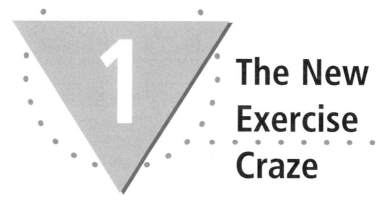

The New Exercise Craze

Everywhere you look people are exercising. Two, three, or four times a week, sometimes more, teens head for the running track, the cycling trail, the rock climbing gym, the skateboard park, or the sports club around the corner. New extreme sports, such as snowboarding, sky surfing, and bicycle stunt riding, have caught many teens' interest. Beyond sports, in a body conscious culture, teens are concerned about physical appearance and body image more than ever. Looking good these days includes stair-climber's thighs, runner's calves, weight-trained upper arms, and rowing machine abs.

Look around you and you will see plenty of these types of body parts on sports stars and celebrities who make looking good seem easy. Check out the stars on *Dawson's Creek* or the hottest singing sensations, like Britney Spears with her athletic antics or Usher and his well-toned physique, and you will see what looking good is supposed to look like.

Many teens who work out do more than just exercise; they have a fitness routine. They plan and schedule their workouts. They identify what part of their body they are going to work on and for how long. They record their workouts in detail, and they count the miles they have run and how many calories they have burned off in the process. For some teens, working out has become an obsession.

SPORTS HIGHLIGHTS

Structuring exercise into your day was not always necessary. When people moved into the cities in the 1800s, the need for structured exercise grew. Before this, people were busy clearing land, plowing fields for crops, and building roads, bridges, and tunnels—difficult work that provided all the exercise a person might need. It was the rise of urban life and middle-class affluence that created so many less strenuous jobs for people.

During the colonial period, sporting activities were fairly simple. Children participated in games and physical activities. Swimming, wrestling, and shooting were popular, as were square dancing and foot races. In the winter in the North, there was skating and sledding.

Organized sports competitions were not common until the middle 1800s. A young Abraham Lincoln was a wrestling champion in New Salem, Illinois, but there were no statewide competitions like today, and Lincoln had to choose another profession. In the mid-1800s, team sports began to appear. Most team sports came from Europe, but basketball and baseball started in the United States and lacrosse was first played by American Indians. Colleges began to organize rowing crews. Team competitions started in rural areas at fairs, at revival meetings, and in cities. As more people played sports, others became excited about watching sports. Players and entrepreneurs started to charge admission fees. Eventually this led to professional sports.

The Civil War (1860-1865) had an impact on the advancement of sports in America. When not fighting in the war, bored soldiers burned off pent-up energy through horseplay and rough-and-tumble play. Some soldiers organized wrestling contests, foot races, and team sports, especially baseball, which helped pass the time between battles.

After the war individual sports and spectator sports became more popular and more organized. Tennis and golf were added as imports from England to the American sports scene. Organizations were started that helped organize sports. The Canoe Association, the National Lawn Tennis Association, and the League of American Wheelmen (bicyclists) were started in the late 1800s. Hockey was imported from Canada in 1893. Sports were not organized at the professional level yet, but athletes started to become teachers and instructors as interest in sports grew and people wanted to participate as well as watch.

Team and individual sports continued to advance into the mid-1900s. Professional sports started to develop as golf and tennis competitions were organized. The first national open golf championship was held in 1894.

RUNNING HITS THE SCENE

A lot has changed in the area of exercise and physical fitness for the amateur and recreational athlete in the last thirty years. What started as jumping jacks in a required physical education course in most public schools in the 1960s became a fitness craze in the 1980s. In the 1980s exercise grew into a favorite national pastime for millions of Americans. Jogging, the popular running sport of many Americans, was a catalyst in popularizing exercise in general.

In 1968 Dr. Kenneth Cooper's book *Aerobics* was published. In it Dr. Cooper suggested that aerobic exercise for twenty minutes three or four days a week was enough exercise to lower the risk of heart disease, improve weight control, and generally help a person feel better. According to Cooper, jogging for twenty minutes three or four times a week was enough exercise to strengthen the heart muscle and decrease the risk of heart attacks. The rate of heart attacks, mostly measured in men, had grown at alarming rates by the 1960s. Cooper's plan appealed to middle-aged businessmen. With busy schedules and limited time for a regular workout routine, jogging fit easily into their schedules. Not only is jogging easy to do, it can be done anywhere—even in hotel rooms for the business traveler. There is no special equipment required to jog except for a good athletic shoe. You do not need to schedule court time, find a partner, or go through the effort to join a sports team to get a workout. Middle-aged men hit the streets running. So did many other recreational athletes.

Running clubs sprang up around the country and

helped to increase its popularity. These clubs spon-
sored special events like the 10K, or ten-kilometer,
run and the 5K, or five-kilometer, run that introduced
so many runners to the sport. Amateur athletes could
participate in these events for fun and for physical fitness. They encouraged each other in their running,
partnered up for weekend runs, and developed a net-
work of running enthusiasts.

Some people became so adamant in their running that they structured most of their time around
it. Bruce Dern, an actor popular during this time,
became a avid runner and kept detailed records of
his mileage, running five to ten miles a day. People
became so involved in their sport that they had little
time for anything but the next running event. For
them running was becoming more than a workout;
it was becoming a compulsion.

Another factor in the increase in running as a popular exercise choice was a book written by Dr. William
Glasser in 1976 called *Positive Addiction.* Glasser
wrote that getting hooked on certain activities, like
running or transcendental meditation, was a beneficial
or positive addiction, unlike addictions to alcohol or
drugs. This was before the damaging effects of exercise addiction had been reported or studied.

Running and jogging continued to grow in popularity. Long distance running hit its peak around
1979. Participation in long distance running events,
such as a marathon, increased tremendously. Three
hundred runners participated in the Boston Marathon
in 1964. In 1979 that number jumped to 7,800 runners. By 1980 a fitness craze was in full spring. A
Gallup poll (a nationally recognized sampling of adult
Americans) indicated that in 1987, 46 percent of all

Americans indicated that they followed some fitness routine, up 20 percent from 1961. Aerobic activities of all kinds were introduced. The aerobics class became a popular choice for structured exercise.

Aerobics classes combine popular dance elements with a vigorous workout routine set to pulsating rock music. Aerobics classes sprang up everywhere—in athletic clubs, recreation centers, college and high school gyms, and even church activity rooms. Teens attended aerobics classes ,too. The high-stepping, arm-pumping exercise with a popular beat appealed to younger people and provided a great workout. And aerobics classes are constantly changing to keep people interested. Steps were added for the step class. The slide allowed you to move from side to side while exercising. Mini-trampolines allowed you to jump into your workout. And kickboxing added a whole new twist to the aerobic routine.

RUNNING IS BIG BUSINESS

The popularity of running meant a business boom as well. Running magazines appeared on newsstands, full of the latest fitness information. New equipment was developed as fast as companies could design new products. Special clothing was designed and soon became necessary for the complete workout—jogging outfits, sports bras, sweatbands, and athletic shoes. Food supplements and sports drinks—from energy bars to Gatorade—filled the shelves at the grocery stores next to snacks and soft drinks and were marketed to the sports enthusiast as nutritional necessities. A fitness industry was born along with the fitness craze.

Sports celebrities like Michael Jordan and Michael Chang were paid huge sums of money to endorse athletic shoes that were designed especially for them. Celebrities were recruited to further the popularity of sports products. Athletic shoes, in particular, became a huge business. The shoes became so expensive that kids robbed other kids at gunpoint to get a pair.

THE LOOK HAS CHANGED

What looks good has changed. Although the perfect man's physique of today is a build with muscles that bulge and a washboard stomach, that was not always the case. In the 1800s and early 1900s, muscles meant that a man had to work for a living. Men of wealth and privilege did not concern themselves with working out or striving to look muscular.

What is considered the perfect shape for girls has also changed over the years. Early in the twentieth century, women wanted to be full figured, soft, and pale. This look implied that they were women with financial resources, not tanned and thin from doing physical work outside or around the home. In the 1940s and 1950s, the era of Marilyn Monroe and Jayne Mansfield, girls girdled themselves to achieve hourglass figures, accentuated by tight cashmere sweaters over pointy brassieres, full poodle skirts with big belts, and little waists. There wasn't a developed tricep or pectoral muscle among them. In the 1960s, thin was in. A British model, Twiggy, became the fashion industry icon.

Twiggy was flat-chested and very thin, with short straight hair parted on the side. Teens starved themselves to get Twiggy's waiflike look.

With the exception of young athletes and sports stars, most girls did not include weight training in their fitness routines until the 1980s. Today girls work out on weight equipment to firm their abs and develop their triceps just as much as boys. Teens today have a new look to model themselves after. The hunk, the workout babe, the fit look is everywhere. They reason if you are not fit, you are not in, or if you are overweight, not interested in sports, or exercise-phobic, there must be something wrong with you. You have to look good to be popular, and today looking good means having no more than 10 percent body fat and muscles that are sculpted to perfection.

TRAINERS AND OTHER EXERCISE GURUS

There are more than 70,000 fitness trainers working in the United States. Many stars and celebrities have personal trainers. Sports stars especially work out with trainers and coaches to maintain optimal fitness. Tara Lipinski, Zina Garrison, and Tiger Woods have coaches and trainers to help them develop their skills and maintain their fitness. Many stars and celebrities have home gyms stocked with the latest in exercise equipment and a trainer to make home visits to help them stay in top form.

A tautly muscled exercise guru of the 1960s, Jack LaLanne, was one of the first exercise celebrities. He started "physical culture" studios, had a TV exercise show, and made guest appearances around the country. With his jumping jacks and calisthenics beamed into people's living rooms via the magic of television, people could exercise along with him. He was a model of fitness, and someone whom you could include in your daily activities.

Jane Fonda went from major film star to fitness advocate with her hugely popular aerobics video in the 1980s. A popular actress in the 1970s, Jane, like many stars, was obsessed with her appearance. Her exercise video sold millions of copies and helped create a market for aerobics workout videos. The message from the video was clear. With a VCR and a television set, you, too, could look as good as Jane Fonda. You did not even have to leave home to do so.

Unfortunately, it is never that simple. Jane Fonda later revealed that her compulsion for fitness included an eating disorder. She had battled bulimia, an eating disorder, for many years. While in her teens and attending boarding school, she started binge eating with friends. She learned that you could eat anything you wanted to as long as you vomited it up, or purged it, afterward. Bingeing and purging are part of the compulsive behavior of people who suffer from bulimia nervosa.

Richard Simmons and Denise Austin are two celebrity exercise enthusiasts of the 1990s. Simmons, once overweight, dieted and exercised his way to fitness. He now conducts seminars and collects fans around the country. Simmons tries to motivate people to lose weight and feel good about themselves in the process. Denise Austin's cable TV exercise show brings workouts from exotic locations into your living room.

Personal trainers became popular in the 1980s.

What started as a luxury for wealthy celebrities and athletes became a necessity for business executives and six-figure-income types who wanted to stay in shape and did not have time to go to a gym. Today many people have personal trainers to help them with their exercise routines. Trainers are available at most sports clubs and fitness centers, and they schedule sessions with clients from the clubs.

Personal trainers are supposed to help keep a person motivated so that he or she will want to work out regularly. Trainers design comprehensive work-out routines to meet a person's unique exercise needs. They build in a variety of different exercises and assist the person as he or she works out. Trainers at sports clubs help clients learn how to use exercise equipment such as weight machines for weight training.

Trainers can cost from as little as $10 an hour to over $150 an hour. They may come to your home or work out with you at the gym. They may even promote exercise adventures, such as backpacking and hiking in the mountains of Nepal, for really ambitious individuals for whom money is no object.

FITNESS GADGETS

Every few months, a new exercise product hits the sports equipment market. This steady stream of gadgets and equipment employs the latest in tech-nological advances and is designed to keep people interested in exercising. Stair steppers, elliptical slides, mini-trampolines, rowing machines, and gravity machines have all been added to the sports equipment market in recent years. Some gadgets

FITNESS AS A NATIONAL GOAL

The physical fitness trend that is so popular today grew out of a fear about the fitness of young Americans for fighting a war. Around the time of the Korean conflict in the 1950s, the results of a national physical fitness test—the Kraus-Weber Test of Muscular Fitness—showed alarming results. It indicated that America's youth were in poor physical condition. If young people were unfit physically, how could they serve in the military?

The President's Council on Youth Fitness was established by President Dwight Eisenhower in 1955 as a result of this information. The name of the council has changed over the years, and its current name is the President's Council of Physical Fitness and Sports. The goal of the council was to set a national standard for fitness for American school children. By the 1960s physical education was a part of almost every child's school day. In the 1980s, celebrity chairpersons such as Arnold Schwarzenegger and Florence Griffith Joyner, were recruited to help popularize physical fitness among young people.

Recess time with games and team sports and playground equipment provided for the physical needs of elementary school children. Secondary schools required physical education classes two to three times a week. The physical education class consisted of a predictable rotation of activities like volleyball, softball, trampoline, and bowling. Classes began with the required calisthenics—jumping jacks, sit-ups, and push-ups—with students lined up in neat rows across the gym dressed in white uniforms and gym shorts. PE, as physical education came to be known, became a dreaded event.

are complicated and high-tech; others are as simple as adding large rubber bands for stretching or using household items like food cans for hand weights. Most of these products are just another high-tech way of doing basic exercises. Although there is improvement in design as technology advances, you do not have to have the latest equipment to get a good workout.

THE CURRENT EXERCISE CRAZE

By the 1980s and the time of the "me" generation, physical fitness was an integral part of the recreational activities of many Americans. It was a hugely popular leisure time activity. No coaches or

PE teachers were required to shout out exercise drills. People were taking it upon themselves to get into shape. Jogging helped popularize fitness with many reluctant nonathlete types. Jogging seemed like an easy way to work out without the intense competitiveness of other sports. Just about anyone could participate in it. It could be practiced anywhere. It did not require a lot of equipment. All you needed was a pair of running shoes.

Streets and parks across America became dotted with a steady stream of joggers. Jogging lanes, running tracks, and athletic clubs sprang up in communities large and small. Today many exercise and fitness activities are popular, from a variety of aerobics and dance-exercise classes to power walking and cycling, from tennis to swing dancing and rock climbing, all the way to extreme sports like snowboarding and sky surfing.

Of course, all this set the stage for an increasing obsession with exercise and fitness and physical appearance. Diet-related illnesses like anorexia and bulimia were becoming household words, and for many teens the new standards of fitness and good looks were unattainable, and the need to constantly exercise seemed to conceal deeper problems of poor self-esteem.

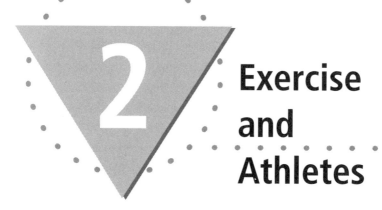

Exercise and Athletes

Professional athletes work out for a living. Most professional athletes have highly structured work-out routines designed to bring them to the optimal level of performance for their particular sport. The success an athlete achieves in a sport can depend on his or her fitness and training program.

THE ELITE ATHLETE

It takes more than talent to rise through the ranks to the elite level of athletic competition. Although you will not get to the elite level without talent, you will not stay there long without a total fitness program and tremendous self-discipline. The athlete who has a complete fitness program is one who cross-trains, who works on various muscle groups through different exercise routines. A complete fitness program prepares an athlete to endure a five-set match in a professional tennis tournament or to race in 90-degree temperature at the national track meet.

Most elite and professional athletes have the help of experts to prepare and develop their skills for competition. Athletes like Tara Lipinski, Andre Agassi, Zina Garrison, and Tiger Woods have a team of experts to assist in their training programs. Fitness trainers, coaches, nutritionists, masseuses, sports physiologists, and sports psychologists are all part of a team of experts who assist the athlete by providing the latest in high-tech training and encouraging the athlete to perform at his or her best. Athletes at this level of competition spend many hours every day training for their sport. Most of their time is structured around the demands of their sport and training programs.

Tara Lipinski started training for her skating career when she was eight years old. She developed a passion for ice-skating after putting on her first pair of ice skates when she was six years old, setting aside the rollerskates that she had used up until the age of three. Tara got up at 3:00 AM so she could get in three skating practice sessions before school. After school it was back to the rink for more training. Tara put her skating ahead of everything else. She wanted to get to the top level of competition, the elite level where she could prove herself and secure a place on the Olympic team. Her goal was to win an Olympic gold medal.

Tara and her mother moved from their home in Texas to Delaware so that Tara could train with a new coach. She left her father, friends, and everything she knew behind her. She left her school and her classmates and had to schedule time for her education with a private tutor. Tara sacrificed many things to pursue her dream. Most teens Tara's age were busy with social activities, friends, church groups, and family. All of that was limited for Tara because of the demands of training for ice-skating competitions. There were many levels of competition to rise through to reach her Olympic goal. For Tara it paid off. She won the gold medal in women's figure skating in the 1998 Winter Olympics when she was only fourteen years old, the youngest skater ever to win the gold medal.

Other young athletes are not so lucky. In those sports where physical appearance is important and body and weight requirements are very strict, like ice-skating, gymnastics, and dancing, many athletes struggle and fail to get to the elite levels of competition. They develop many problems from the demands of training and competition, including injuries, eating disorders, and exercise addictions.

EXERCISE ADDICTION AND ELITE COMPETITION

Although skating consumes her life, Tara Lipinski appears to be enjoying her sport and has many years of professional skating ahead of her. It seems as if she is in control of her skating career and her life. Other athletes face problems and challenges not easy to overcome.

Athletes who compete at the highest elite levels of competition have training requirements that, to the observer, may look like excessive exercise. Dr. Rick Aberman, a sports psychologist in Minneapolis, Minnesota, says that you have to look at the demands of a sport when evaluating whether a person's exercise routine has become obsessive. For example, Aberman cites the case of a college athlete who was training for cross country track competitions and running 140 miles a week. The athlete was told to decrease the amount of miles he was running. But Aberman points out that this much training is required for competing at the intercollegiate level.

Kari had been training for a chance to go to the Olympics in gymnastics since kindergarten. Her parents were thrilled that she wanted to be an Olympic athlete. They signed her up for gymnastics classes when she was five years old, after she had watched her sister compete in a college meet. Kari said she wanted to be like Dominique Dawes and Shannon Miller. She read every article and book she could find about them and other Olympic gymnasts.

As Kari advanced in her sport, her parents decided that she needed to train with the best coaches at the best training camp available. They enrolled her in an elite gymnastics training camp where Coach Kawalski worked. Not everyone was allowed to train there and Kari was thrilled to be selected for Coach Kawalski's camp. This was the camp where Kristie Lerner, another Olympic gold medalist, had trained.

Training was difficult and demanding. Long workouts seven days a week put a stress on Kari and her body. Kari did not always feel like training. Some days she wanted to take a day off. At other times she was exhausted from the strenuous workouts and begged to stay home. Many times she had so many aches and pains that she did not think she could endure another day of training. But Kari's parents encouraged her to continue, saying that she would get used to the workouts—plus she had come this far already. As much as she dreaded going to her training sessions some days, she hated to miss one. Coach Kawalski scolded the gymnasts if they missed a session. He said they were weaklings and not cut out for the top levels of competition. If a gymnast missed a session, to make up for it, she would have to train longer the next day.

By the time of the regional qualifying round, the hard work was beginning to pay off. Kari took second in the overall individual events. She was thrilled with the silver and so was her coach. Kari overheard Coach Kawalski brag to his assistant coach that she was "the next Kristie Lerner." Kari was about to burst with pride at being compared to Kristie, one of the best gymnasts in the world, when she heard Kawalski add, "If she'd just drop a few pounds, she might have a chance to make the Olympic team before she's too old."

Kari was devastated. Although Coach Kawalski had teased her about her appetite before, he had kidded many of the gymnasts about their weight. Some of the gymnasts starved themselves. They limited their food intake to one meal a day. Sometimes they did not eat anything the day before a big meet. But Kari had always shrugged off the coach's jokes and ate what she wanted. After working out for eight hours a day, Kari was always hungry.

This time she did not shrug it off. It hurt her to hear that the coach thought she was overweight.

She wanted to make it to the Olympics no matter what it took. The next day Kari cut her calorie intake in half, to no more than 600 calories. She measured out what she could eat carefully, cutting her food into small portions and counting up the calories of every bite of food she ate. She skipped breakfast so that she would not be tempted to overeat later in the day. Sometimes the temptation was too strong and she stuffed herself after a long day of training. Pizza and cookies were her weaknesses, and she kept a stash of cookies in her room and hid frozen pizza behind the juice in the freezer.

After a binge Kari was always bummed out and sick to her stomach. But she couldn't help herself. She was starving half the time as it was. The 600-calorie diet was torture. One day she complained to Rachel, her teammate, about how she was struggling to lose weight and feared that she wouldn't make the Olympic team.

"I've got to lose ten pounds or I'll never make the team. But I'm always starving after workouts," said Kari. "I can't stop stuffing my face when I get home."

"Just throw it up," said Rachel.

"What?" asked Kari. She was not sure she heard correctly.

"Make yourself puke. I do it all the time," said Rachel. "How do you think I keep my weight down every day?"

"Gross," said Kari. "No way. I can't stand puking. I wouldn't be able to do it anyway."

"Just stick your finger down your throat and up it comes," said Rachel. "Nothing to it."

The idea of sticking her finger down her throat grossed Kari out. What could be worse than making yourself vomit. But she had to lose weight. The next competition was only a month away. That night after dinner, when she had eaten a huge plateful of spaghetti at her best friend's house, she excused herself and went into the bathroom. She stuck her finger down her throat and made herself vomit.

Kari felt sick and ashamed afterward, but it had worked. The next day she had lost a pound instead of gaining one back. Kari had discovered a new way to deal with her weight issues. Whenever Kari stuffed herself, she made herself purge by vomiting. It was a trick the other girls at the gym were using all the time, she discovered. Within a week she had lost five pounds, even though she continued to binge regularly. Soon Kari came to feel bloated and disgusted with herself if she did not make herself throw up after eating. Her throat was sore and her stomach hurt most of the time but she could not stop purging even if she wanted to. She was hooked into a cycle of bingeing and purging that was starting to wear on her health. She felt tired most of the time and she was starting to get more injuries during workouts. Even Coach Kawalski was yelling at her, calling her skinny and telling her she had no energy in her workout routines.

Both professional and amateur athletes can develop eating disorders and become compulsive exercisers, addicted to their workout routines. The demands of training and competing at this level are intense. The weight requirements of sports like gymnastics, wrestling, ice-skating, and dancing make it that much more difficult. Jockeys also frequently struggle with eating disorders and other addictions because of the demands of their sport. Runners, cyclists, swimmers, and others can develop eating disorders or become addicted to exercising.

Top gymnasts are small and lightweight. In a 1994 University of Utah study of elite gymnasts, those training for the Olympics, 59 percent admitted to some form of eating disorder. Cathy Rigby, a former Olympic gymnast, struggled with bulimia and anorexia nervosa for twelve years. Zina Garrison, a professional tennis player, has battled anorexia and bulimia, and former tennis professional Carling Bassett-Seguso battled anorexia for a time.

Ballet dancers, usually considered artists rather than athletes, have some of the most finely developed physiques of any performer. They twist and contort their bodies to form the perfect arabesque or pirouette on the tips of their toes. At the professional level, competition is keen. Prima ballerinas, those who play the leading roles, are thin and frail looking. Many dancers are intimidated into thinness by the demands of these principal roles and by their teachers and choreographers. In an effort to stay thin, many dancers develop eating disorders. After the anorexia-related death of professional ballet dancer Heidi Guenther, the spotlight has been turned on the training techniques of these dancers. Schools have started to add nutritionists to their staffs and to instruct their dancers on the dangers of anorexia nervosa and bulimia. Dancers who are dangerously thin are put on alert to gain weight and are followed closely by the staff.

Wrestlers who must wrestle below their normal weight face the same problems. Often coaches and trainers are unrelenting in their demands for weights far below what is normal for the athletes' height and body type. Wrestlers may go through starving rituals to make their weight before a big match. William "Refrigerator" Perry, defensive lineman for the Philadelphia Eagles, has also struggled with compulsive overeating.

3 Exercise and Addiction

What is your exercise routine? How long have you had it? When do you exercise? Where? Why? Most people who exercise regularly do so for fitness, to stay in shape and look good. But people get other benefits from exercise. Although physical fitness, or getting into shape, is the most common reason people work out, some people exercise for social contacts, to spend time with friends and family, to improve their mood, or to manage stress.

It was Friday night and Josh did not have a date. Most of the kids Josh hung out with were going to a dance. Josh hated to go to things like that without a date. He felt like everyone was looking at him.

Josh hung around the house for a while, watched some ESPN, and played with the dog. Then he started to feel agitated. He kept thinking of how Stephanie, a major babe and star on the girls' basketball team, had turned him down for a date to the dance. The more he thought about it, the angrier he got. Josh grabbed his gym bag and his sports clothes out of the closet. As soon as he started throwing shorts and shoes into the gym bag, he felt better. He was out the door and headed for the rec center in record time, slamming the door shut behind him.

At the rec center Josh ran into Terry and Martin, his workout buddies. Every day after school they met in the weight room to work on their weight training. They high-fived each other and then joked around with Lisa, the girl at the front desk. On the way to the weight room Terry started to give Josh a hard time.

"Hey, Josh. Where's Stephanie?" Terry asked, punching Josh in the arm.

"Who wants to know?" replied Josh, punching Terry back.

"Who wants to know? We want to know, man. I thought you had a hot date tonight. At least that's what you said."

Josh flushed red with embarrassment. He looked around the weight room to see if anyone was listening. But he was lucky. Since it was Friday night, most kids who usually worked out at the center were at the dance.

"Yeah, well, I don't see your big date around either," Josh shot back, grabbing the weight off of the bar.

"Okay, studs, to your corners," said Martin, putting his hands out between them like a boxing referee.

"What do you say to a game of challenge?"

Martin said, trying to change the subject. He eased onto the weight bench next to Josh and checked the weights at the end of the bar.

"You're on," said Josh, giving the weight bar an extra pump before setting it back on the rack. Josh figured he would win the challenge tonight for sure, as pumped as he was. There was no way he would tell Terry and Martin that he had asked Stephanie to the dance but she had turned him down.

For some people, working out is more than a way to stay fit. It is a way to socialize—to hang out with old friends and make new ones. For others, exercising is a way to work off stress—to relax and get away from the pressures of home and school. Exercise is helpful in these ways. It can be a healthy way to take a break and get back your perspective on things. Difficulties occur when you use exercise to avoid problems instead of dealing with them.

Mindy slammed the door to her bedroom. She jumped on the bed with a huff and buried her head in her hands. Every time she had a fight with her mom she wanted to get as far away from home as she could. But now that she was grounded, her room was as far as she could go. "I can't wait to get out of here," she thought.

Mindy had just had a huge blowup with her mom. It was another fight about Jess, her boyfriend. Mindy was fighting with her mom about him more and more. Mindy knew her mother did not approve of him, although at first she did not say anything. When Mindy first started dating him, her mom would just nod as Mindy talked about him. But lately, every time she mentioned she was going out with Jess, her mom had that look in her eyes, like she got when her dad said he had to work late or her grandmother criticized her mom's cooking.

Now her mom was complaining because Mindy wanted to stay home and go to State College instead of going to school in Oregon like she had been planning to do. Jess was going to State and she wanted to go there, too. Besides, you would think her Mom would be happy because of all the money they would save on tuition. The more she thought about it, the madder she got. Her mother did not understand how much Jess meant to her.

"You're throwing your whole future away!" her mother screamed at Mindy when she announced her new college plans.

Mindy jumped off the bed, grabbed her tennis racket, and ran down the stairs in a huff. If she hurried she could get in an hour's practice on her serve before it got dark.

"Where do you think you're going?" Mindy's mom yelled as Mindy ran down the stairs two steps at a time.

"Out!" Mindy yelled, the front door slamming behind her.

Mindy practiced her serve until her shoulders hurt and she could barely throw the ball into the air. But she did not care. The harder she hit the ball, the better she felt.

DIET AND EXERCISE

Exercise is recommended by nutritionists and physicians as part of a healthy diet and weight control program. It helps control appetite, makes you feel good about yourself and your body, and burns calories in the process.

Ask any teen what the number one concern of most teenage girls is and he or she will likely tell you diet and weight. Teenage boys, too, are concerned about weight and body image more than ever before. Most teens want to look good.

Many teens use exercise as a means of weight control. Pick up any teen magazine and the cover is splashed with the latest diet craze and workout routine in big bold letters. Inside will be a section devoted entirely to diet and exercise. It will include tips on how to lose weight faster and easier. Articles like "Lose Twenty Pounds in Twenty-Four Days" or "How to Firm Up Flabby Thighs and Sagging Buttocks" will promise quick fixes and miracle changes. The photos that go with the articles show models with perfect bodies who must have become thin by following the diet and doing the exercises. Page after page of advertisements in the magazine offer diet drinks, exercise equipment, and weight control programs, all available to help you lose weight fast. The message is clear: If you want to look good, this product will make it happen.

Burning calories, however, should not be the main focus of your exercise routine. This is where problems occur, when you exercise exclusively to burn calories or lose weight. If you use exercise to purge yourself of calories, only to tell yourself that it is now okay to have that extra slice of cake because you can work it off the next day, you could be headed for an exercise addiction.

BENEFITS OF EXERCISE

You need some form of exercise every day to maintain a healthy body. In the "good old days," exercise did not have to be structured into your day. Most of your day involved exercise in some form, whether it was from walking—because it was the only way to get around—or because of the hard work that was part of everyday life before machines did so many things for us. People got health benefits from their routine daily activities.

Today most people have to structure exercise into their daily lives. Living in a service economy with many modern technologies, most Americans do not have to use a lot of physical energy to earn their living. Today all you have to do is push a button on your remote control to turn on your television and your VCR, or use the cell phone in your pocket to order in pizza. Your heart does not have to pump very hard, your lungs do not have to get completely aerated, and your legs do not have to stretch to get through the day and accomplish what is required of you.

To get the health benefits of physical activity, people must structure exercise into their daily and weekly activities. There are many physical and emotional benefits of exercise. Exercise provides a cardiovascular workout. It raises the heart rate and strengthens the heart, as well as other muscles.

Physical Benefits of Exercise:

⊙ It improves muscle tone.

⊙ It increases energy reserves.

⊙ It lowers body fat.

⊙ It slows the resting pulse rate.

⊙ It lowers blood pressure.

⊙ It lowers cholesterol.

⊙ It relieves muscular stress.

⊙ It promotes restful sleep.

⊙ It promotes regularity of bowel movements.

Psychological Benefits of Exercise:

⊙ It builds self-esteem.

⊙ It relieves stress.

⊙ It promotes a sense of well-being and balance.

⊙ It provides social opportunities.

⊙ It encourages setting and achieving of goals.

⊙ It promotes a healthy outlet for competitive energy.

WHEN EXERCISE GOES TOO FAR

Exercise is good for you. It is recommended by physicians and nutritionists as a way to build a healthy body. It does not seem possible that something so good for you could be harmful to you when overused or abused. But it can. You can use exercise to avoid facing problems. You can exercise compulsively as part of an eating disorder to purge yourself of calories. You can become so involved in the competitive nature of a sport that you overexercise, get repeated injuries, and become exhausted from your workouts instead of feeling refreshed and energized. You can become addicted to exercise psychologically or physiologically.

Compulsive exercise is exercise that has gone beyond a normal, healthy activity. Exercise addiction has many similarities to other addictions, such as alcohol or drug abuse, shopping, or gambling. The person who exercises compulsively becomes preoccupied with exercising and spends a lot of time thinking about and planning his or her workouts. The compulsive exerciser is so involved in exercise activity that he or she excludes other activities. When not exercising, the compulsive exerciser experiences withdrawal symptoms. He or she feels agitated, angry, depressed, guilty about not exercising, fearful about gaining weight, or worried about losing the training progress that has been made. What exactly happens when you exercise too much, when you become obsessed with exercise?

Kim has had a weight problem all her life. During Kim's childhood, her dad called her his little pumpkin, round and sweet. By the time she was in her teens, Kim hated the nickname. She flashed red with embarrassment every time her dad called her that, a name that used to make her feel special.

She had tried every diet that came out in the teen magazines. They worked for a week or two, then she got tired of them and binged for three days. But Kim had learned a new trick. One day she overheard some girls talking in the locker room. A group of girls from the dance squad were talking about how they lose weight. Sherry, the squad leader, said you could eat anything you wanted as long as you threw it up afterward. At first Kim was grossed out. But she thought that if it worked for Sherry, she might as well give it a try. The next day Kim stuffed herself with pizza and chocolate cake from her brother's birthday party. She stuck her finger down her throat and made herself throw up. It was gross, but it worked. She could eat what she wanted because she would vomit it all up afterward.

Kim started to lose weight. She added exercise to her diet routine. It helped her to burn off calories and control her appetite. Now that she was losing weight it was easier to stick to her diet. Kim's mom was proud of her progress and gave her a membership to the health club for her birthday. For the first time Kim started to feel good about her body. She started to wear tighter clothing, not the usually baggy jeans and big T-shirts. She went to the health club regularly. The more she exercised, the better she felt. She started to exercise compulsively, going to two or three exercise classes a day. Soon she felt agitated and disgusted with herself if she missed a *day of exercise. She was certain she would gain back the weight she had worked so hard to lose.*

Kim started putting exercise ahead of other activities. She built her entire day around her exercise schedule. She started keeping a journal to record her workouts and the food she ate each day. She carefully calculated the calories she took in and the calories she burned off by exercising. Kim was hooked. She could not miss a day of exercise without feeling anxious and fearful about not exercising.

WHO CAN BECOME ADDICTED TO EXERCISE?

Anyone can become addicted to exercise, but some people are more at risk than others. According to Dr. Carl Chan, a physician in the Sports Medicine Center at the Mayo Clinic in Rochester, Minnesota, the people most susceptible to developing an exercise addiction are those who channel all of their energy into a certain sport and who have had a degree of attainment in that sport. Certain sports lend themselves to exercise addictions. Running, bicycling, aerobic dancing, and other aerobic activities like swimming are sports that put people at risk more than others. But people can become addicted to almost any exercise routine at the psychological level, whether the sport is basketball, weight lifting, golf, or tennis.

People are more likely to become addicted to exercise if they prefer individual sports over team sports. They also tend to be self-coached, that is, they do not have someone working with them as a trainer or coach who can be objective about how much they are exercising. The person who is addicted to exercise will continue to work out even when injured, fatigued, or ill. Exercise addicts avoid going to the doctor for injuries, and when they do go, it is only for a quick fix so that they can continue with the exercise routine and not to care for injuries to their bodies.

A person is more likely to become addicted to exercise if he or she limits activity to one sport exclusively. Although many recreational and professional athletes cross-train to develop a total fitness program, the exercise addict resists this. Even when advised to do so, he or she will ignore these suggestions and focus exclusively on his or her preferred sport.

People are more likely to become addicted to exercise if they use all their nonschool and non-working time to exercise. Exercise addicts focus exclusively on their sport and their workouts instead of getting involved in after-school activities, joining clubs or organizations, getting a part-time job, volunteering in the community, or developing talents and interests.

CHECK YOURSELF

Here is an exercise addiction checklist. If you answer yes to several of these questions, it could indicate that you have an addiction to exercise.

⊙ Do you see yourself as fat or out of shape even when others say you look good?

⊙ Are you trying to create a "perfect" body through exercise?

⊙ Do you think constantly about exercising?

⊙ Do you alter your daily schedule to make time for exercise?

⊙ Do you pursue one sport or workout routine exclusively?

⊙ Have you lost interest in your preferred sport but continue to overexercise anyway?

⊙ Do you prefer to exercise alone?

⊙ Are there many stresses and problems in your family?

⊙ Have you had repeated injuries related to exercising?

- Even when injured, do you continue to exercise?

- If a doctor tells you to stop exercising for a time, do you ignore that advice and continue to exercise?

- When recommended to cross-train, do you disregard that advice and continue with your preferred workout?

- Do you keep detailed records of your exercise workouts?

- Has exercising caused you to lose weight beyond what is normal for your height and body type?

- Do others suggest that you exercise too much?

- Do you have difficulty sleeping when you are unable to exercise for a day?

- When you cannot exercise, do you feel anxious, agitated, guilty, or depressed?

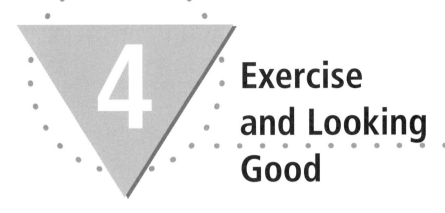

Exercise and Looking Good

Image is everything. You are bombarded with that message every day. Flip through the pages of any teen magazine and you see teens in the photos and advertisements who are the image of perfection—flawless with their toned bodies and their perfect skin. Television shows and movies are full of beautiful people, too—actors and actresses with spectacular bodies who look like they were born that way. Commercial advertisements show beautiful people taking risks and doing cool and daring things. The message is clear: Buy these products and you, too, can look this good and have this fabulous lifestyle.

Most teenage girls are concerned about diet and weight. Teenage boys, more than ever before, want to look good and improve their body image. It is what most of you talk about over lunch or in between classes or after school. And most of the talking you do about yourself is negative.

"I look so fat in these jeans."

"Do these platforms make my legs look big?"

"Did you see the arms on Mark McGwire? I wish I had arms like that."

"I hate my hair like this. It makes my cheeks look huge."

The message sent by American culture is that image—your outside appearance—is important in many ways. Most people tend to make quick judgments about others because of what they look like. Studies suggest that people who are considered attractive tend to get better jobs and are promoted more often. Many teens believe that if you look a certain way, you are guaranteed popularity. You may even do better in school and get along better with your teachers and coaches. If you are concerned about your image and what others think about how you look, as most teens are, there is a good reason. No wonder you go around checking yourself in the mirror all the time.

THE IMAGE BUSINESS

Many businesses and industries promote their products and services by associating them with images of what looks good and is appealing to potential customers. For example, the fashion industry depends almost entirely on images, and likes to suggest that a new clothing line, a new eyeglass frame, or a new style of shoe will give you not only a certain look but an appropriate lifestyle. The tobacco, soft drink, and sporting goods industries all promote an image that suggests how cool you can be if you use their products. Every year hundreds of millions of dollars are spent on research, test marketing, and advertising to promote a look or image that businesses hope you will want to copy. These "image industries" encourage the belief that image is everything.

The image industries are always coming up with "the latest look" to promote new products. The ad campaigns that are created for these companies try to set trends or invent fads for a new product line. The fashion industry creates a new image of what looks good every fashion season. Fashion-conscious teens cannot wait for the spring or fall magazines to come out so they can see what the latest fashion trends are. The new looks keep the consumer interested in buying new products.

Tobacco companies create images to make smoking look cool. The Joe Camel ads of the 1980s were accused of appealing directly to teens with Joe Camel's funky antiestablishment look. Consumer groups protested and the ads were taken off the market. Athletic apparel companies use celebrity endorsements to help promote their products. When Michael Jordan was king of the basketball courts, who wouldn't want to be like him and play as well as he did by buying a pair of Nike shoes?

A particular look and appeal for a product is carefully researched to see what teens like and what they will buy. Many ads are also designed to appeal to teens' insecurities. Other companies, rather than trying to set trends themselves, try to follow fads that teens are setting themselves. These companies spend thousands of dollars on research to see what teens think is "hot" and what interests them. Teen Research Unlimited of

Chicago, a market research firm, has hired a panel of teens to see what they like and do not like. The teens are able to express their opinions through focus groups—sitting around a conference table and sharing ideas about different products. By participating in focus groups, the teens provide the research company with valuable information about the teen consumer.

Ironically, the latest research suggests that teens today are resisting the images companies are trying to create for them and instead are coming up with their own ideas about what is hip or in style. This is why you now see more quirky ads that suggest a product is cool because it goes against the establishment, and more that poke fun at adults.

WHAT DO YOU FIND ATTRACTIVE?

What a person finds attractive varies from individual to individual. Although popular imagination says that a guy should be tall, dark, and handsome and that a girl should be big-breasted with a tiny waist and long shapely legs, very few real people match those ideals. These images became part of our belief about what is appealing after years of exposure to books and magazines and movies showing what the perfect guy and the perfect girl were supposed to look like. Even today, the heroes and heroines of popular children's videos are more shapely than ever. The characters look like they have been on the stair-climber all day getting into shape before putting on their medieval clothes. Everyone has been influenced by the fitness craze.

The fact is that in spite of advertising and image

making, most people are attracted to different types of looks just as they are attracted to different personalities. But it becomes hard to know what you are really attracted to because you are so bombarded every day with images that you lose the ability to judge for yourself.

Do you see a hairstyle you like on someone else and want to have your hair cut the same way? Do you want to have that outfit your best friend wore to school? Most teens look to others for models of what they want to look like. When you see an athlete you admire advertising a certain type of athletic shoe, you may buy that shoe because you want to be like that athlete. Or maybe an athlete wears his or her hair a certain way, like Michelle Kwan, and you want to have your hair cut the same way.

Look around you. Who do you consider attractive? Why? What is it about him or her that you find attractive? Is it his or her face? His or her hair? His or her body? What is it about his or her body that is attractive? Does he or she look like someone you know? Someone in the media? Is this person someone you know? What is he or she really like as a person? Would he or she make a good friend or is he or she just nice to look at? Pretend that you don't know the person. Would you find the person attractive if you didn't know him or her?

If you are really honest about what you find attractive, not what some magazine, television show, or advertisement suggests is attractive, you may find that you really like something totally different. First impressions are hard to ignore but sometimes they are misleading. If you examine what you find attractive, you may discover that you are attracted to the way a person smiles, the way a person helps someone by offering to carry his or her notebooks, or by the friendly way that person asks how your day is going. You may find yourself responding not to a packaged image, but a real person.

THE BUSINESS OF IMAGE MAKING

Sports stars on the tennis court or the golf course are wearing clothes covered with logos these days. They are paid huge amounts of money to be celebrity endorsers. Celebrity endorsers pitch products on television commercials, on billboards, and in print advertisements all the time. Michael Jordan wore Nike athletic shoes when he played for the NBA because he was a paid Nike endorser. Tiger Woods endorses products for several companies who want to capitalize on the young golf pro's appeal. Tennis celebrity endorsers are usually the latest grand slam winners. You do not see sports stars as celebrity endorsers unless they are winning regularly in their sport.

Image making is a huge business. Sports stars are under a great deal of pressure to rise to the level of competition where they will be awarded contracts for product endorsements. Once at that level, the pressure is even greater to stay there. Amateur athletes in particular feel this pressure and push hard to make it to the Olympics because it is only after winning a medal that there is a chance of being asked to sign on for product endorsements. In fact, only a gold medal usually brings these endorsement offers, and only certain Olympic medalists are considered marketable. For example, even if you win a gold medal in wrestling, weight lifting, or swimming, you probably will not get product endorsements unless you win several medals in different events. On the other hand, medal winners in the "appearance" sports—figure skating and gymnastics—almost always get product endorsements.

The movie business is based on images, too. Movies are full of beautiful people who are paid huge salaries and pampered daily to keep a perfect image. Although many stars are talented actors, often their careers are made or broken because of what they look like. If a star adds a few pounds, changes a hairstyle or loses his hair, his career could be affected by it. The star may lose popularity or not get as many good roles. Contracts for actors and actresses in long-running television series often require them to keep the same hair style and general appearance for the duration of the show.

Stars and celebrities have large staffs of specialists to help them look good. They have personal trainers, nutritionists, chefs, personal shoppers, masseuses or masseurs, and even plastic surgeons all working to help them maintain the perfect image. It is a lot easier to look good when you have all those people pampering you and providing support. Even with all this help, however, many stars and celebrities struggle with their weight and self-image.

Occasionally you read in the tabloids about a

star who is struggling to lose weight at some spa or who is battling anorexia. Stars are not very forth-coming about the problems they have with weight control, particularly with eating disorders, out of fear of a bad reaction from the public. But some do. Talk show host Oprah Winfrey talks openly about her problems with weight gain. Jane Fonda admit-ted that she struggled with bulimia for years.

WHAT'S HOT AND WHAT'S NOT

Images of how we should look are always changing. In the 1960s, the British fashion model Twiggy pop-ularized the pencil-thin look. Not only was Twiggy thin, she was flat-chested, a new look for the rebel-lious 1960s. Television shows like *Suddenly Susan* and *NewsRadio* made red hair for women popular again in the 1990s. Close-fitting mini tops, short skirts, platform shoes, bell-bottom pants, and polyester—all a fashion throwback to the 1970s—made it big again in the 1990s. The guys on *Dawson's Creek* and *Party of Five* all look like they just came from the gym.

What products we buy to enhance our image also change over time. In the early 1990s, Levi's, Converse, and Nike were hugely popular. In the late 1990s, it is Tommy Hilfiger, Mudd, and Paris Blues. Product placement in movies and televi-sion shows also helps to promote them. When you see a star sipping a certain cola with a recogniz-able label, that is product placement. The recent increase in stars smoking in movies may be due to the influence of the tobacco industry. Top fash-ion designers give stars tuxedos and gowns to wear to premier events so that their designs will be associated with the beautiful people. These industries know that you are influenced by what you see stars doing and wearing.

BODY IMAGE

For many years girls grew up with the saying "You can't be too rich or too thin." Today the saying would probably be "You can't be too fit or too thin." The message today is that you cannot devote enough time to staying in shape. The sculpted physical appearance that comes from pumping iron and working out is what many teens strive for. Muscles are sculpted to perfect tone by repetitions on the weight machines. Every muscle is worked on, pumped, toned, and stretched to perfection. And it is not just the guys spending time in the gym.

Most girls did not want to have muscles before the fitness craze hit in the 1980s. Muscles were for guys. Only men needed muscles anyway. They were the strong ones, the ones with the jobs that required physical labor, the ones who did the tough work around the house. For girls, unless they were athletes, in which case muscles were acceptable and working out to get them was required, they did not want to pump up. Girls did not want to look like a guy. Girls wanted to look feminine, soft, and curved.

All that started to change with the fitness craze. Girls started hitting the weight machines as much as the boys. The shape of the female body changed. Cindy Crawford, a supermodel in the 1980s and 1990s, helped make working out and looking fit popular. She was athletic, not the usual waiflike model that girls and women were used to seeing.

IT'S WHAT'S INSIDE THAT COUNTS

With all the emphasis on the way you look, it is hard to believe sayings like "It's what's inside that counts" or "You can't judge a book by its cover." People do tend to judge others based on what they look like. Most people are not aware that they are making these judgments. They think that they do not like someone because of an annoying habit or personality trait, but subconsciously they may be judging someone's appearance. Many teens worry about how others see them or whether they are considered attractive. Image, or the way you look, has a lot to do with the way you feel about yourself.

Amy picked up the latest issue of her favorite fashion magazine and started thumbing through the pages. Beautiful models in summer fashions with perfect tans and perfect bodies leapt off the pages. The more she looked, the more depressed she got. It was close to spring break and Amy was supposed to go to the beach with her best friend's family. But she hadn't had her swimsuit on for months, not since the beach party in September before school started. Amy felt like a blimp. She had been eating whatever she wanted all winter. And she had skimped on her workout routine.

Amy pulled up her sweater and looked at her stomach. Her stomach pushed against the snap on her jeans, hanging over the waist in little rolls. She jumped off the bed and stood in front of the full-length mirror on the closet door. She turned from side to side. Her thighs looked huge, too, she thought, as she pulled on the fabric of her jeans. She had to squeeze into her jeans that morning and struggled to get them snapped shut.

Amy started to panic. Spring break was less than a month away. She had never leave the beach house if she looked like this. Amy turned to face the mirror head on. "Fat, fat, fat," she told herself. She went to her dresser and pulled her bathing suit out of a drawer. It was a bikini she had gotten last summer when she was at her best weight in years, orange with yellow flecks. She had bought it with her baby-sitting money. Amy held it against herself as she looked in the mirror. "No way. I'm huge," she moaned.

Amy sucked her stomach in and tried to hold it in but she couldn't. Her stomach pushed out over her waistband. "Gross," she thought. "What am I going to do?" Amy picked up the magazine again. "How to Lose Ten Pounds in Ten Days" it said in bold black letters on the front cover. "Ten pounds in ten days, I can do that," she thought. "Last time I fasted to lose weight, I lost five pounds in a week. This should be easy," thought Amy. She flipped the magazine open to the section on diets and exercise.

Most teens are concerned with their image, says Dr. Deborah Wright, an adolescent therapist. She agrees that what teens see in the media has a lot to do with how they feel about themselves. But most images are impossible to live up to. The way you look is a combination of genes and environment, but mostly genes. You inherit your physical features from your parents. If you have a big nose, chances are your dad or mom does, too. If your thighs turn in when you walk, unlike the perfectly shaped model's thighs you see in the magazines, you may have inherited them.

Some of these physical attributes can be improved upon or even changed. Cosmetic surgery has become more common at younger ages. But it is a drastic measure that is usually unnecessary. Physicians are careful to screen patients, particularly teens, to determine who really needs cosmetic surgery and why they are requesting it. According to the American Society of Plastic and Reconstructive Surgeons, 3 percent of all cosmetic surgeries in 1994 were for patients eighteen years old or younger. In 1998 it was 2 percent. The top five procedures in 1994 were nose reshaping, ear surgery, breast reduction for males, breast augmentation for females, and liposuction.

Other aspects of your appearance can be improved through diet and exercise. You can exercise and tone muscles that seem flabby, stomachs that bulge, and arms that need strengthening. You can improve your image, but you cannot change your basic bone structure, or feet that seem too large or too small, or how thick or thin your hair is, or how far apart your eyes are.

Furthermore, changing the way you look is not going to make you happy if other things are bothering you. It will not give you more friends or make you successful. If you have some physical feature that is really troublesome to you, changing it in some way can improve your self-esteem, but not for long if you do not feel good about yourself inside. Diet and exercise to tone your body will not make you perfect. Perfection should never be the goal of exercise. But if exercise will make you feel good about yourself and accept yourself for the unique individual that you are, that is a worthwhile and attainable goal.

5 How Do You Feel About Yourself?

How do you feel about yourself? Do you think you are smart, talented, skilled at computers, good with people, a good athlete? Or do you think that you are stupid, a loser, a klutz, or a person with no special skills or talents? How do you feel about yourself when you look in the mirror? Do you like what you see? Do you think you have a nice face, good hair, a friendly smile? Or do you pick yourself apart, looking at each feature and examining what is wrong with it? Is your nose too big? Does your chin recede into your face and make you look like you don't have one? If you are like most teens, whatever you see in the mirror is never good enough.

The way you feel about yourself is called your self-esteem. It affects you in many different ways. How successful you might become, how well you get along with others, who you choose for your friends, and who you are attracted to and want to date are all affected by your self-esteem. The way

53

you see yourself is called your self-image. Your self-image is shaped not by what you see when you look in the mirror, but by what you think you see. Do you like the shape of your legs or the way your arms look? Do you see a large person or a thin one in the mirror? Do you see someone who needs to lose a few pounds or someone who is at an ideal weight?

The way you see yourself and how you feel about your body can affect you in many ways. If you have a good self-image, you accept the way you look. Although there may be things you would like to change, you think you look okay. When you have a good self-image you walk confidently down the hallways at school. You think you look hot in your new sports jacket. When you shop for clothes, you don't freak out when you see yourself in the dressing room mirrors. Even swimwear does not create a crisis. No matter what shape or size you are, you are comfortable with your appearance.

It takes most teens a long time to feel okay about the way they look. When you have a poor self-image, you do not like the way you look. No matter what you look like, it is not good enough. You are always trying to change things. If your hair looks okay, you do not like the way your pants fit. If your skin has cleared up, you wish you had smaller hands. There is always something about your appearance that could be improved on.

WHAT IS SELF-ESTEEM?

Self-esteem starts the day you are born. You might

look at it as a kind of savings account that starts when you are very young—something that you carry with you all the time. There are many things that go into this savings account. The way people take care of you when you are little goes into the savings account. Do they respond to your needs quickly or wait a while? Do they encourage you to grow and try new things, or do they pamper you and do everything for you? What do they tell you about yourself and your feelings? Do they call you a crybaby when you fall down and scrape your knee and start to cry? Or do they get you a bandage and try to make it better? If you are afraid of the dark, convinced there is a monster lurking in the closet, do they get a flashlight and help you look for the monster and chase it away? Or do they tell you there are no such things as monsters and that you should stop being so afraid?

What people say to you as you grow up also goes into your savings account. If people tell you nice things about yourself, these expressions of affection go into your savings account and nourish you years later. If they say bad things to you, if they tell you that you are no good, that you are stupid, that you are clumsy, that you look ugly, you will have bad things in your savings account, and these expressions of disappointment could haunt you in the future.

The people who are closest to you—your parents, your brothers and sisters, your grand-parents, your friends—put many things into your savings account because you are around them most of all. They have more opportunities to add things to your savings account, and you care very much about what they do or say.

Other life experiences also add or subtract from your self-esteem. How you do in school is a big factor. If you perform well on tests, get good grades on your homework, get along with your teachers and your classmates, you are storing up a lot of self-confidence. If you are coordinated and can quickly learn the skills it takes to master a new sports activity, that will boost your self-esteem. But if you struggle to learn new things, if you fumble and fall while learning to play catch and kids tease you about being slow and clumsy, that will have a negative effect on your feelings about yourself.

Years later, when you are learning a new skill at your job or a new dance at a rehearsal, you draw from your savings account. You don't give up when things become difficult. You give yourself time to learn and practice the new skill and you don't berate yourself or say negative things to yourself.

Matt was excited. Today was the day that his big brother, John, was going to teach him how to ride a skateboard. He had been look-ing forward to this day all week. As soon as John got home from his job at the grocery store, he was going to take Matt to the skating park.

Matt had gotten a new skateboard for his sixth birthday, and he could not wait to learn how to ride it. His brother, John, was one of the best skateboarders in town and had won sev-eral competitions.

"Let's go, Squirt," said John as soon as he walked in the door. "Squirt" was the name he had called Matt since Matt was a little boy. It gave Matt a warm feeling inside when John called him that.

"Cool, let's go," said Matt, grabbing his board.

"You boys be careful!" yelled their mom from the kitchen.

"Aren't we always?" yelled John over his shoulder as they headed out the door.

When they got to the park it was packed with kids racing up and down the curves of the cement walls. The shining colors of the skateboards glimmered in the sun. The whirl and scrap and squeal of skating filled the air.

"You ready, Squirt?" asked John as he set his board on one of the ledges. He strapped on his knee pads and elbow pads and then put his helmet on and strapped it under his chin.

"Ready," said Matt, setting his skateboard down beside John's and putting on his protective pads, too. Matt started to step onto the board.

"Whoa, buddy," said John. "Not so fast. First, I want you to watch me." John headed up the ramp.

John pushed off with his right foot and then stepped onto the board heading down the ramp. He whooshed up one side of the wall and down another one, weaving his way around other skaters. Soon he whooshed to a stop inches away from Matt's feet.

"What d'ya think?" asked John.

"Awesome, let's go," said Matt, starting to climb on his board.

"Wait a minute. Let's start over here." John headed toward a level strip of concrete, gently guiding Matt by the shoulder.

"Come on," said Matt. "I want to do the cool stuff, not this baby stuff."

"I had to start with this baby stuff, too," said John.

John instructed Matt on how to push off to get a running start and how to balance his weight in the middle of the board. When Matt bumped into another kid and tumbled to the hard concrete, John was right there to help him up.

"You okay, Squirt?"

"Yeah, I'm fine. Darn, I was going good."

"You're doing great, kid. That's the way to use your arms to balance. Let's try it over here where it's not so crowded."

As they walked over to a less crowded area, Matt heard a kid yelling, "Watch out!" Then he saw another kid about his age tumble to the ground. Another kid went rushing over to him screaming at him. "What's wrong with you, you klutz? Dad's right. You can't do any-thing right."

The kid brushed off a scraped knee as blood trickled down his leg. Matt saw a tear run down his cheek. Matt felt bad for him. He reached up and grabbed John's hand. He was glad his big brother did not talk to him like that.

It takes time to learn new skills. Matt was learning that you have to master the fundamentals before you can do the more difficult tasks. With John as his teacher, he learned that even someone who is very good at a sport had to start as a beginner. John showed him that you do not get good at something right away. It takes practice and patience. Being patient as you learn something is better than berating yourself about it. Others should not berate you either. Matt's brother had built up his self-esteem by projecting positive feelings about learning something new. The other kid at the park was not so lucky and may suffer from the effects of his brother's attitude for years to come.

As you have new experiences, your reservoir of self-esteem increases. You draw from this reservoir years later in ways that you are usually not aware of. In the future, when Matt tries to learn a new sport or skill, he will learn to keep trying and he will not feel bad about himself if he cannot do it right away. But he will not necessarily remember that this positive attitude came about because years ago his brother was patient and encouraging when he taught him new things.

The way you feel about yourself changes from day to day. Sometimes you feel good about yourself and your self-esteem is high. At other times, you may not have such a good day and your self-esteem is lower. Nobody feels good about him- or herself all the time. You have good hair days and bad hair days. You feel more competent some days than others. But you should feel good about yourself most of the time.

SELF-IMAGE

Self-image, or the way you see yourself and how you feel about your body, starts at an early age. If people started telling you when you were four that you were chunky, you started to see yourself that way. Even as you grow and change, you continue to see yourself as fat.

While growing up you are often compared to others in your family. Family members may tell you that you have your father's eyes or that you walk just like your brother. Sometimes it makes you feel good to be compared to others. If you like Grandpa, you feel good about being like him. But eventually you want to be acknowledged for who you are. Like most teens, you want to be unique. Everybody wants to be recognized for their own unique looks and qualities. You are a unique individual, unlike anybody else. Even when you are a twin or a member of a large family, your personality and experiences make you different from your siblings.

While others are busy comparing you to family members, you are busy comparing yourself to peers, movie stars, rock stars, sports stars, and models. It is hard to like the way you look when there are so many others to measure up to. Most teens look at themselves and see only what they don't like about themselves. Even if they have beautiful skin and a flashing smile, they will see eyes that are too far apart, hips that are too narrow, and feet that are too big. They see parts of themselves instead of looking at themselves as a whole person. People tend to focus on what is "wrong" with their looks instead of what they like about themselves. They want to be perfect.

If you like what you see when you look at yourself, you have a positive self-image. You may work on the way you look. You may exercise, watch what you eat, and wear certain clothes, but mostly you feel good about your body. You have confidence in yourself and your self-esteem is high. If you do not like what you see, if your body is never good enough, you have a poor self-image. You are always trying to change something about your body or the way you look. You may go on diets constantly, change your hairstyle every week, or exercise excessively to improve the way you look.

Although American culture attaches great importance to good looks and perfect bodies, what most people consider attractive in others is their attitude. Self-confidence, a sense of style, humor, kindness, generosity—these are qualities that make a person appear attractive to others. An attitude of self-acceptance is a very attractive quality.

Look around you. When you see people who act like they are cool, like they have it all together, they may seem appealing and attractive. But look at them closely. They probably don't have the model-perfect looks that you see in magazines. Maybe their ears are a little bigger than some, or their lips are fuller, or they have skinny legs, but they don't seem to care. They seem to like themselves just the way they are.

People who tease you about your looks are usually insecure about their own looks. What people say about you has more to do with how they see themselves than how they see you. It is not easy to ignore hurtful comments about your looks. The pain these comments cause can last a long time.

6 Growing Up

S ometime between the ages of ten and sixteen for girls and between eleven and sixteen for boys, puberty begins. Puberty is something all teenagers go through eventually. For most teens, puberty is a time of confusion and change. Your body is changing and growing in new ways. Your emotions are changing, too, causing mood swings and intense, confused feelings. With so many things changing during puberty, both physically and emotionally, it is no wonder many teens feel anxious and disoriented during this time.

WHAT EXACTLY IS PUBERTY?

Puberty is the process of changing physically and emotionally as you become an adult. The word comes from the Latin *pubes,* which means "adult." The process starts when a tiny gland at the base of your brain, the pituitary gland, switches on and tells various organs in the body to start making hormones. These hormones create major physical changes in the size and shape of your body, after which you become an adult with the ability to sexually reproduce.

The exact age that puberty begins is different for everyone. When puberty begins for each person depends on his or her genes and environment. Knowing when your mom or dad, or an older brother or sister, went through puberty will be a clue to tell you when you will start puberty. What your parents and grandparents look like will have some influence on the outcome of the physical changes you experience. They may be tall or short, have thick hair or thin, have big feet or small, and you will likely have a combination of these traits. This information is transmitted in the genes you inherited from your parents.

Your environment can also affect the changes you go through in puberty. The onset of these changes can be affected by your diet or by exceptional situations that create a lot of stress for you. "Everybody in my family was the shortest in their class until they hit their senior year. Then they grew three inches," said Nick. That is Nick's genes at work. "I didn't get my period until I was sixteen. All my friends had gotten theirs," said Joan. "I felt like a freak. But my gymnastics coach said it's not unusual to start your period later when you are in serious training for gymnastics." That is Joan's environment at work.

FOR GIRLS

Sometime between the ages of ten and sixteen, girls will start puberty. This process of becoming an adult means that you are developing a woman's body. You are going through many physical changes, including the hormonal changes that allow you to become pregnant. When you start menstruating, this really signals that puberty has begun.

You develop breasts and your hips fill out. Your face gets fuller and longer. The composition of your skin changes. Your face or back may break out as your skin produces more oil. You get more hair on your body. The hair on your arms and legs thickens and you grow hair under your arms and over your genital area.

Physical Changes for Girls During Puberty:

⊙ Bones in the face mature and the face looks more "grown up."

⊙ Breasts and nipples grow larger and fuller.

⊙ Ovaries enlarge inside the pelvis.

⊙ Thighs get rounder.

⊙ Appetite increases and more sleep is needed.

⊙ Arms, hands, legs, and feet grow bigger and longer.

⊙ Skin becomes oily.

⊙ Hair grows under the arms.

⊙ Waist narrows and hips widen.

⊙ Hair grows around vulva.

⊙ A person thinks about sex more often.

⊙ Normal sticky, whitish discharge from vagina.

⊙ Menstruation begins.

⊙ Body sweats and smells.

⊙ Height and weight increase as muscle and bone mass increase.

The changes of puberty are caused by hormones in your body, especially the sex hormones estrogen, progesterone, and testosterone. Boys and girls produce all three of these hormones but in different amounts.

Girls produce greater amounts of estrogen and progesterone. These hormones act on the ovaries to produce an egg every month. You get your period when the egg is not fertilized and the lining of the uterus is shed. If you have unprotected sexual intercourse around the time that the egg is produced—in a process called ovulation—and the egg is fertilized by the male sperm, you get pregnant. What many girls do not know is that even before you get your first period, your body could be starting to make these changes, and you could be fertile and get pregnant. Girls who train rigorously for sports or who run a lot or work out vigorously, will sometimes miss periods. Girls who have eating disorders may experience a delayed puberty.

A girl's final growth spurt generally occurs with the onset of menstruation. But intense physical training and low food intake can delay menstruation. If a girl does not begin menstruation until she is older, her final period of growth may never occur, or it may occur to a lesser degree. It was only after she retired at the age of twenty-five that Olympic medalist Kathy Johnson started menstruating. She grew a full inch when she was twenty-eight.

Girls grow breasts because of the sex hormones. The size of the breasts is mostly determined by the genes you inherited from your parents and grandparents. Many girls feel self-conscious as they go through these changes. They compare themselves to others around them. If your breasts are large, you may feel awkward and self-conscious. If your breasts are small or you are slow to develop, you may feel insecure, wondering when you will get breasts like your friends. It is not unusual to start puberty before your friends have or to be the last one to go through the physical changes of puberty.

The sex hormones cause other changes as well. You grow hair under the arms and around the sex organs. The hair on your arms and legs thickens. Hormones also cause you to develop more muscle mass and bone mass. This causes you to get taller and gain weight. Many times girls do not understand these physical changes. As they gain weight, they do not understand that this is a normal part of puberty. They try to diet or exercise to control the weight gain. Sometimes they become anorexic during this time, unconsciously trying to stop the changes of puberty.

FOR BOYS

For boys, puberty usually begins between the ages of eleven and sixteen. Growing into a man means many physical changes. You grow more hair on your body. Your voice changes as your larynx grows. Your voice may jump an octave while you are talking to a girl you have a crush on, causing you major embarrassment. Your face matures as it gets wider and more angular. Your skin gets oilier ,and you may get acne. You become wider across the shoulders. You develop more bone mass and muscle mass, and you get taller and gain weight. You can bench press more weight.

Physical Changes for Boys During Puberty:

⊙ The face matures as bones in the face grow.

⊙ Shoulders and chest grow wider.

⊙ Soft hair, which becomes course and curly, grows around the penis.

⊙ The penis grows larger and longer and the scrotum darkens.

⊙ Arms, hands, legs, and feet grow bigger and longer.

⊙ Appetite increases and more sleep is needed.

⊙ The voice "breaks" as the larynx enlarges.

⊙ Hair grows in the armpits and on the chest, arms, and legs.

⊙ Testes grow larger and fuller and become sensitive.

⊙ A person thinks more about sex.

⊙ Wet dreams and ejaculations start to occur as sperm are produced.

⊙ The body sweats more and smells.

⊙ The skin becomes oily and pimply.

⊙ Height and weight increase as muscle and bone mass increase.

Boys produce the three sex hormones, testosterone, estrogen, and progesterone, during puberty just like girls do. But in boys the pituitary gland tells the testes to make more of the hormone testosterone, the male sex hormone. This means that you can produce sperm. Sperm are mixed with a fluid called semen. If you have unprotected sex after reaching this stage of puberty, you could impregnate a girl. If semen is ejaculated during sexual intercourse and reaches the girl's egg in the uterus, a pregnancy could result.

The sex hormones produce other changes, too. Hair growth increases. You grow facial hair. The hair on your arms and legs thickens, and hair grows on the genital area and under the arms, and sometimes on your back.

As you gain weight and build muscle mass, you may grow breast tissue. For some boys, this is terribly embarrassing. Genetics plays a role in how you develop physically, and you may have inherited this tendency from a family member. If it bothers you, talk to someone about it like your parents, a physician, a school nurse, or counselor. There are options available to you, including diet, exercise, and cosmetic surgery.

THOSE SEXUAL FEELINGS

Eric was well prepared for his book report. He had practiced the night before, reading the book report out loud to his sister, Lorraine. She gave him the thumbs up after he finished, and he felt certain to ace it.

Eric hated to speak in front of the class. But he knew it was something he needed to work on. His speech teacher suggested that he could reduce his anxiety about speaking in front of the class by being prepared: know the book from cover to cover, write the book report well ahead of time instead of the night before, and practice, practice, practice. It was working. The more Eric practiced giving the report, the more confident he felt that it would go well.

When he looked in the mirror the next morning and saw the pimple that had popped out on his chin, Eric groaned. "Geez, just what I need, a big ol' zit." He grabbed some of his sister's tinted acne cream and covered it up as much as he could.

In English class, the teacher called on the students alphabetically. Eric's heart raced every time Mr. Williams said a name. When he got to the Ls, Eric thought his heart would pop out of his chest, it was pumping so hard. His palms were sweating, and he felt tight in the chest. "Calm down, calm down," Eric said to himself. "You're just anxious about giving the report. Everything's cool. You're ready, my man," he added for confidence. It was helping. Eric relaxed a little.

"Eric Larson," the teacher said from the front of the room.

Eric jumped out of his desk and bolted to the front of the class. He took his book report out of his back pocket, took a deep breath, and began.

"Lord of the Flies *is set on an island . . ."*

Just then the hallway door opened to his left. In walked Jennifer, the hottest girl in class.

"Excuse me. Sorry I'm late," Jennifer said, brushing in front of Eric as she put a late slip on the teacher's desk.

Eric thought he would die right there. As she brushed in front of him, Eric flushed and felt strangely excited. He flashed red in embarrassment. Eric felt certain that the whole class was looking at him and could tell that he had an erection. He thought Jimmy was laughing at him from the back of the room as he leaned across his desk to whisper something to Cary.

He might as well be standing in front of everybody naked, he felt so embarrassed. He wanted to bolt from the room and never return. But he took a deep breath and contin-ued talking. He started to feel better as he talked. The practice had paid off, and he finally got into the swing of things. He began to relax.

Sexual feelings can be wonderful, stimulating, and exciting. Or they can come at what seems like the worst time and be embarrassing, scary, or even shameful. Sexual feelings, like other feelings, are unpredictable. But the more you learn about your feelings, what they are and how to respond to them, the more manageable they become.

During puberty, hormonal changes create a growing sexual awareness as you mature and develop. Sexual awareness means that you feel sexual desire and are attracted to others sexually. These sexual feelings combine with your other feelings to create a state of emotional flux, in which your moods change unpredictably.

What you learned about your body as a growing child can affect the way you feel about your developing body as a young adult. If you learned that your body was a source of pride, something to feel good about and enjoy, then you learned to take care of your body, to value and nurture it. If you learned that your body was something to be covered up and hidden, that bodily functions like sweating and urinating were disgusting, that sex and masturbation were bad or dirty, then you learned shameful feelings about your body.

Your growing sexual awareness means that you find boys or girls attractive now. Before you found boys or girls disgusting or stupid and you did not want anything to do with them. You teased them on the playground and did not want to play with them. Although you probably had crushes on a boy or girl in your class, you didn't really spend much time with them, like you do with your regular friends.

As sexual awareness increases, you think about sex more. You become aroused and fantasize about being with someone you are attracted to. It can be fun to fantasize about someone. The crushes you have on the guys or girls around you—or on movie stars, sports stars, and rock stars—can grow into a full-blown obsession. But sometimes sexual feelings can be overwhelming. Instead of creating excitement, they create a feeling of confusion or fear. You don't like these feelings. You may try to stuff yourself with food to make them go away. Or you may turn your sexual energies into exercise and sports.

Channeling your sexual energy into other activities can be healthy. Part of becoming an adult is learning to manage your sexual feelings and to act responsibly. Acting out sexually is dangerous. For many people, exercise and sports are a healthy way to work off sexual energy. But for some, exercise can be a way to hide sexual feelings, to deny that you have these feelings. Exercise can become a compulsive way to deal with sexual feelings or any feelings that make you uncomfortable.

Sexual feelings can lead to sexual contact. Being sexual is the closest you can be to someone. It is a form of intimacy that can be very threatening or scary. Some people block out their feelings either consciously or unconsciously while sexually involved. They may have sexual contact, but they deny there were any feelings involved. "It was just sex," they say, denying that there was any intimate or emotional contact. People who approach sex in this way are depriving themselves of a full sexual experience and can hurt others emotionally.

Sexual awareness and desire continue to grow during puberty. It is strongest for boys during their teens and early twenties. Women reach the peak of sexual desire in their thirties, toward the end of their reproductive years.

TOO MANY CHANGES

All the physical changes of puberty do not happen at the same time. You may get taller before you gain muscle mass, so you look skinny or narrow in the shoulders. Your feet may grow before the rest of you does, and they may seem huge, sticking out in front of you. You may grow as much as an inch overnight. This is called a growth spurt. You go to school the next day in pants that stop at the ankles because they are suddenly too short. You may get your second set of teeth before your face changes, making you feel like you are all teeth for a while. Your face may break out in a rage of pimples, and no one seems to understand how awful that makes you feel. They say things like "Don't worry. It's just hormonal. Your skin will clear up soon." That does not seem promising. The physical changes of puberty can make you feel awkward and clumsy.

The emotional changes that come with puberty can seem overwhelming. One minute you feel like an adult, and the next you want to be a kid again, hanging out with your dog in your room. The hormones that are affecting your body affect your moods, too.

It does not seem possible that these things are normal, but they are. It is normal to feel clumsy. It is normal to feel as if the only thing people see when they look at you are your zits. It is normal to feel moody and depressed, as if the whole world is against you. It is normal to pull away from your family and want to do more things on your own. Many things change as you go through puberty in the process of becoming an adult.

Although you used to feel self-confident and did not let things bother you, now you are not sure about anything. When you are called on in class you feel self-conscious, as if you are going to say the wrong thing. You worry about your appearance and whether girls or guys find you attractive. You worry about how you are developing physically. Most teens worry about the size and shape of their genitals and how they are developing. Are they too big, too small, the right shape? These fears are a natural part of maturing physically.

Things are changing around you as you go through puberty, too. For example, people may treat you differently. Your parents may give you more responsibilities. They may expect you to do more around the house or to help with your brothers and sisters. They may want you to talk to them more about your problems, or they may even talk to you more about their problems. Your parents may expect you to get a job and contribute to household expenses.

You used to have a good relationship with your parents. You could talk to them about anything. Now they don't seem to understand you anymore. You fight about the littlest things: what you wear, what time to be in, who your friends are. The fighting seems endless. You would rather tell your best friend your deepest troubles than confide in your parents.

Part of puberty is growing away from your parents. As you develop into an adult physically, you also want to become more independent. You want to spend time with your friends, not at family gatherings. Parents do not always understand your need for independence, or they may simply not be able to acknowledge that you are becoming an adult. Sometimes you are not sure how you feel about this either.

Teachers and other school personnel may treat you differently, too. Teachers may give you more homework with a greater degree of difficulty. They may push you to excel and to win competitions and awards. Coaches may expect more from you as a team member. If you are on an athletic team, you may take more of a leadership role as you mature. As an individual athlete, you may be expected to reach higher levels of performance. The more people expect of you, the more pressure you feel to do well. This can be very stressful. Sometimes adults don't realize how stressful these new responsibilities are.

No matter how you are changing and growing during puberty, you are not alone. All teens go through the many changes of puberty eventually. If you are having a difficult time with puberty, talk about it with your parents, a counselor, the school nurse, or your physician. Sometimes these changes can seem overwhelming, and a teen may develop an eating disorder or an exercise addiction to cope with puberty.

7 Patterns of Addiction

When Tamara was in the eighth grade, she took up running. Her dad was a runner and spent his evenings after work running five miles around the neighborhood park. One day he told Tamara to get her running shoes and join him. Tamara started to run with her dad every day after school.

At first, Tamara jogged only a few blocks with her dad and then waved him on as he headed off for his five-mile run around the park. But Tamara found she liked running. It made her feel good. She felt energized and clear-headed after she ran. It had the unexpected benefit of helping her lose a couple of pounds. Tamara decided to increase her distance until she could run the full five miles with her dad. Tamara expanded her workout routine. She did stretches before running and worked out to her mom's aerobics tapes every day. Each week she added another mile to her jogging distance.

Within two months she was running the full five miles with her dad without difficulty.

Tamara's dad was proud of her. He boasted to the family that one day she would win the Boston Marathon. Tamara's mom, too, was encouraging her and telling her how good she looked now that she had dropped a few pounds. Besides making her feel good, Tamara enjoyed running with her dad. She set new goals for herself, planning to run in the city marathon by the end of the summer.

Tamara worked hard at her new sport. It really boosted her self-esteem to work at something that made her feel good. She increased her distance until she could run ten miles easily, then fifteen miles, three times a week. The more time she put into running, the more difficult it was to keep up with her other activities. She started to cut back on the time spent on homework assignments, no longer turning in the work to the teacher on time as she had before. Her mom was starting to complain that Tamara wasn't getting her chores done every day. She shrugged it off. She wasn't willing to miss a day of training. If she did, she felt guilty and bloated.

One day Tamara's parents had a huge fight, and her dad moved out. Tamara was devastated. She knew that her parents had been having problems but she didn't think that it was anything serious. That day she ran until she couldn't run any farther, collapsing on the side of the road clutching her side. She dragged herself home and took a long shower, trying to soothe her tired muscles.

Tamara's dad tried to keep their after-school running dates until he moved across town. He called her and told her that it was just too difficult to make it to her house after work. Tamara told herself she didn't care. She set new goals for herself and ran every chance she could. The added exercise was tough on Tamara's body. Shooting pains raced up her calves when she ran. One day when Tamara came home from running in severe pain, her mother insisted that she see a doctor.

The doctor told Tamara that she had stress fractures and that she had to stop running for two weeks. Tamara protested that it would throw off her training schedule. But the doctor said that there would be more serious problems if she didn't take some time off. Tamara tried to relax and lay off the running. But by the second day her legs started to twitch and she felt edgy and depressed. Tamara was certain that she would lose the progress she had made in her training. Tamara taped her shins and started to run the next day.

A week before the marathon, Tamara got the flu. She stopped training for one day but was depressed and guilt-ridden that she had to miss that day of training. The next day she lied to her mom and said that her fever was gone even though it was more than 101 degrees. Tamara got her running shoes and headed outside. By the following week, Tamara's legs ached and she was exhausted. On the day of the marathon, she had to add extra tape to her shins and drink Pepto-Bismol to keep from vomiting. She made it to the start of the race. She collapsed at the six-

teenth mile and had to be rushed to the hospital because of dehydration and a hip injury.

WHAT IS AN ADDICTION?

Maybe you have a friend who drinks too much alcohol or who has a problem with drugs. Most people think of an addiction as a problem with substances like alcohol or drugs. But you can become addicted to substances other than mind-altering drugs and to certain behaviors or activities as well. For example, you can become addicted to caffeine, shopping, gambling, or exercising.

Many people are addicted to the caffeine that is in coffee and soda and must drink them every day. They cannot get started in the morning without a dose of caffeine, and they get headaches if they do not have a cup of coffee or a cola drink sometime during the day. Many teens drink colas and other drinks that have caffeine in them, like Mountain Dew or Surge. Although research has not identified the exact effects of caffeine conclusively— some studies say it is addictive, others suggest that it is not addictive—there are millions of people who cannot go for a day without a caffeinated beverage. These people experience the physical symptoms of withdrawal if they stop drinking caffeinated beverages—nervousness, severe headaches, and sluggishness.

You can also become addicted to certain activities or behaviors. People who are compulsive shoppers have closets filled with clothing that they never wear, many pieces with the tags still on them. You can get such a kick out of shopping that you get hooked on it. It gives you a high or a rush similar to a chemical high. You find that you have to shop. You feel anxious and depressed if you cannot go shopping, so you shop to relieve these feelings. After the high of shopping comes the low, the guilt and depression about spending too much money and buying things that aren't really needed.

Some people become addicted to exercise. It may not seem possible to become addicted to something that is good for you, but you can. The point is that if you exercise compulsively, you will lose its benefits. Like other activities or substances that are used in excess and abused, too much exercise can be bad for you.

CHECK YOURSELF

Here are some questions to ask yourself about how much you exercise and whether your attitude toward exercise is a healthy one.

1. Do you think about exercise a lot?

2. Do you spend most of your free time involved in a sporting activity?

3. Do you no longer enjoy exercising or participating in a particular sport but force yourself to do it anyway?

4. Do you have repeated injuries from exercising but keep exercising anyway?

5. Do you feel anxious, agitated, depressed, disgusted with yourself, fat, and bloated if you cannot exercise?

6. Do you exercise to purge yourself of calories?

7. Do you keep detailed records of your workouts?

8. Do you think about your body a lot and exercise to try to perfect your body's appearance?

Addiction is getting hooked on something so strongly that you become dependent on it. You can become addicted to a chemical substance, such as a drug or alcohol, because it gives you a temporary feeling of well-being. A physical activity like exercise can create a similar effect by releasing endorphins in the brain that produce a sense of pleasure.

Exercises such as running are reported to have this effect on some people. The runner's high is a feeling of euphoria you get after you have run a certain distance. Endorphins, chemicals with pain-relieving properties released by the brain, are supposed to cause this feeling, although the mechanism is not clearly understood. Workout routines and other types of sports can have this effect, too. Any aerobic activity that increases the heart rate for a sustained period of time, about twenty minutes or more, can have this effect.

People participate in sports such as golf, tennis, or swimming to such an extent that they become hooked on them, too. They become upset and agitated when they miss their scheduled playing time. This is a psychological addiction. The person becomes addicted to the excitement of competition and the release of stress they experience when playing.

Dr. Rick Aberman, a sports psychologist, occasionally sees people in his practice who are addicted to exercise. "You have to see what happens when they can't exercise," says Aberman about the exercise addict. Compulsive exercisers will experience withdrawal. Some indicators of withdrawal include increased agitation, anger, or depression when unable to exercise, and resistance to suggestions to take time away from exercising even if the person is injured. The exercise addict will also resist suggestions to cross-train if he or she is focused exclusively on one sport. Often the first time parents have a clue about what is going on with a teen exercise addict is when that person is forced to stop exercising.

STAGES OF ADDICTION

Usually you do not become addicted to an activity or a chemical substance right away. It happens over time. Addiction to alcohol or drugs progresses through stages. A person gets progressively more dependent the more he or she uses drugs or alcohol. Alcohol and drug addiction start with recreational use, then progress to abuse, and finally to dependence.

The same can be said for exercise addiction. People addicted to exercise usually start exercising for recreational reasons. They may have different reasons for exercising initially—to get into shape, to lose weight, to have a social activity. But what starts as a recreational activity can become an addiction. Eventually such people abuse exercise by training when they are injured or using exercise to purge their bodies of calories. They stretch their bodies beyond what is healthy and work until they are fatigued and exhausted. They are no longer getting physical benefits out of the exercise, but they continue to exercise anyway. With every workout they become stiff, sore, and out of breath.

Eventually they become dependent on exercise. They experience withdrawal symptoms when they are not exercising. They feel anxious, angry, depressed, guilty, and restless when they cannot exercise. People addicted to exercise can feel withdrawal symptoms even when they think they are not going to be able to exercise.

Tolerance

As people exercise, they build up muscle strength and endurance. This means they are developing physical tolerance for the activity. To get more benefit from their exercise, they will have to increase the level of activity.

Todd started weight lifting to increase his chances of making the football team. He started to bench-press 150 pounds. Soon he had to add more weight to get the same effect from the workout.

Jenny was a cyclist. She used bike riding to relax after a busy day. By the time she rode downtown and back, a distance of about four miles, she usually felt like the stress of the day was gone. Lately, though, she still felt edgy by the time she got home. She had to add another mile to her bike ride to unwind from the stress of the day.

Denial

Randy loved to play golf. Every afternoon he was out on the golf course as soon as the last bell rang at school so he could get in nine holes before dusk. In the summer he even got a job at the country club to be able to play golf whenever he had the chance. Randy's girlfriend teased him that she never saw him anymore because he was always at the golf course. She said golf was more important to him than she was. Randy protested, saying that he had to make some money for college that fall. But the next day when it rained and Randy had to cancel his golf game, he was angry and agitated. He snapped at his girlfriend when she called to see if he wanted to go to a movie instead. After the movie when the sun peaked out, Randy gave his girlfriend some excuse about having to get home early. He grabbed his clubs and headed for the driving range so he could hit some golf balls and the day wouldn't be a total waste.

Randy was in denial about his addiction to playing golf. He would never admit that he had to get to the golf course every day or that he felt anxious and angry about it. People in denial do not admit how dependent they are on a sport or exercise routine. Many times people in denial will not acknowledge the effect that injuries are having on their bodies. Even though they are experiencing repeated injuries and yet continue to exercise, they deny that they are hooked on exercising.

Craving

Tasha loved to take dance classes. It made her feel good about her body and herself when she finished her workout. Dance classes were very difficult, especially her ballet classes. After a fifty-minute class she was drenched in sweat and completely drained, but she felt great inside. When her teacher went on vacation for two weeks, Tasha found that she craved the good feelings she got from her dance class. She decided to run extra miles to get the same feeling that she got from her dance classes. Tasha found she had to keep adding miles to get the same effect. She ran five, six, seven miles a day to get the high she got from dancing. Tasha couldn't wait until her teacher got back from vacation. She decided to go to a health club and take some aerobics classes to add to her running routine until her dance classes started up again.

Tasha was craving the feelings she got from her dance class. It became so strong that she had to find a substitute activity—running and aerobics classes—to get the same feeling she got from her ballet classes. The intense workout from a ballet class may release endorphins and produce a plea-surable effect similar to the runner's high. Tasha was craving this high. Some studies suggest that the release of these chemicals may create changes in the brain that cause cravings. A crav-ing is an intense desire or need for something that produces a pleasurable sensation. It causes you to repeat an activity or behavior over and over to get the pleasurable feeling. Eventually, however, you build up a tolerance, and you must increase the level of activity or the amount of chemicals you take to get the same effect. In time, you pursue the activity or chemical just to rid yourself of the withdrawal symptoms.

Withdrawal

People who are addicted to alcohol or drugs experience intense physical reactions when they stop using the addictive substance. Sweating, tremors, shakiness, and nausea are physical symptoms of withdrawal from chemical use. Other symptoms are emotional, such as depression, anxiety, agitation, and irritability.

People who are addicted to exercise can experience withdrawal symptoms when they are not exercising. Withdrawal symptoms include physical symptoms such as twitching or cramping muscles, stiffness or soreness, or fatigue. They also include emotional symptoms such as depression, irritability, anxiety, and self-deprecation.

WHAT HAPPENS WHEN YOU BECOME ADDICTED TO EXERCISE?

People exercise for different reasons. Some people exercise for the health benefits. Exercising every day is part of their lifestyle as much as having fresh fruits and vegetables every day. Exercise is good for you. It provides a cardiovascular workout, making your heart muscles pump blood through your body at an increased rate. It provides extra oxygen to your body's cells and aerates the lungs. It tones and strengthens muscles and builds bone mass. But too much exercise can destroy the very things you are trying to strengthen and build.

People who are addicted to exercise can damage their muscles and bones to such an extent that they require surgery for hip replacements or repair of torn ligaments and cartilage. Social relationships may suffer, and problems with work and school become more serious.

In the book *Hooked on Exercise,* the authors suggest that there are different kinds of exercisers. (See the For Further Reading section at the back of this book.) There is the avoidance exerciser, the obsessive-compulsive exerciser, the body image problem exerciser, the eating disorder exerciser, and the person who exercises to manage depression and anxiety.

According to the authors, the avoidance exerciser uses exercise to avoid problems. This exerciser avoids situations or activities because he or she fears failure. The person may have experienced failure associated with some situation or activity sometime in the past, or he or she expects to fail in the future. Exercising allows the person to feel competent and in control.

The obsessive-compulsive exerciser uses exercise to control anxiety by setting rigid and well-structured exercise schedules. This type of person is goal-driven and a perfectionist. He or she also does not like spontaneity or surprises. While exercising, these people know what will happen for a set period of time. They plan their workouts in detail and do not vary from their plans. Should something occur that upsets their workout schedule, they criticize them-selves harshly and are anxious and guilt-ridden.

The body image problem exerciser uses exer-cise as a way to improve self-acceptance and self-worth. These exercisers look at exercise as a way to improve their bodies so that they can be happy or liked by others. When a body image problem exer-ciser cannot exercise, he or she feels unattractive and worthless. Such people have an unrealistic fear of what will happen if they cannot exercise for a day or a week. They fear that they will turn flabby and be totally out of shape.

The eating disorder exerciser uses exercise to control food intake or burn off calories. The person with an eating disorder who is anorexic uses exer-cise to burn off additional calories. The bulimic per-son uses exercise to purge himself or herself of food from binge eating or before binge eating occurs.

Exercise addicts with anxiety and depression become dependent on exercise to control their moods. Exercise can be an effective way to boost one's mood and feelings of self-esteem. But the person who becomes addicted to exercise eventu-ally loses this benefit. An hour or two after exercis-ing, the person may feel "blah" again. For mood exercisers, increasing tolerance to exercise will increase the amount of time and effort required for the exercise to boost the person's mood, leading to exercise abuse and the risk of injury.

CROSS-ADDICTION TO EXERCISE

Exercise is a healthy alternative for people who have problems with addictions to drugs or alcohol.

Exercise is often recommended as a way for a person who is addicted to drugs or alcohol to add some healthy alternatives to a self-destructive lifestyle.

Occasionally, however, a person who is exercising as part of a program to treat alcohol or drug addiction transfers those addictive tendencies to exercise. For example, a person with an addiction to alcohol may take up running as a healthy alternative and a way to structure some of his or her free time. But if that person never worked on any of the issues that were contributing to the addiction in the first place—difficulties getting along with peers or family members—he or she may focus exclusively on running. Whenever any problems come up at school or at home, problems that the addictive personality should confront, that person goes running instead. Soon this person is hooked on running as a way to feel good and avoid problems. The person has transferred his or her addiction to exercise.

8 Eating Disorders

Many people who have had eating disorders developed these conditions when they were in their teens if not earlier. Teens are very vulnerable to developing eating disorders. In a body-conscious culture, you worry about your weight and your diet more than anything else. As your body grows and develops, you compare yourself to your friends, your peers, and other teens, especially those you see in the media. You are constantly wondering, "Am I thin enough, tall enough, attractive enough?"

In a national survey of 8,000 fifth to ninth-graders, only 45 percent of girls, ages ten to fourteen, and 59 percent of boys of the same age group responded "often true" or "very often true" to the statement "I feel good about my body." According to the National Association of Anorexia Nervosa and Associated Disorders, 86 percent of those with eating disorders developed food-related problems by their twentieth birthdays. Of this number, 10 percent say their problems started at or before age ten, and 33 percent experienced problems between the ages of eleven and fifteen.

Eating disorders include anorexia nervosa, a form of self-starvation or severe limiting of food intake due to fear of gaining weight, and bulimia, which involves a cycle of binge eating followed by purging of food. Other types of problems, often called disordered eating, include compulsive overeating, the use of diuretics or laxatives, and compulsive dieting.

One survey of youth reports that 67 percent of males between the ages of ten and fourteen say that controlling their weight is very important to them. Other studies report that the main concern of high school and college boys is to gain strength and muscle definition, with as many as 53 percent expressing a desire to lose weight. The rate of anorexia nervosa and bulimia in males, however, is believed to be underreported. It is not considered "manly" for a male to have an eating disorder. But this is changing as more males admit that they have a problem with eating disorders.

Many athletes, particularly in "appearance" sports (such as gymnastics, figure skating, and dancing) where weight requirements are strictly defined, have suffered from eating disorders at one time or another. Christy Henrich, an elite gymnast from Kansas City, died from complications of an eating disorder when she was only twenty-two years old. Heidi Guenther, a professional ballet dancer with the Boston Ballet, died from complications of an eating disorder when she was the same age.

According to one expert working with eating disorders, 20 to 30 percent of individuals with eating disorders are athletes. The American College of Sports Medicine estimates that up to 62 percent of female athletes participating in certain sports may have eating disorders. In a University of Washington study of 182 female college athletes in 1992, 32 percent practiced some form of disordered eating. For college gymnasts, that figure jumps to 62 percent, almost double. However, about 18 percent of the general female population suffers from some form of disordered eating. American gymnastics officials claim that the sport of gymnastics does not cause eating disorders. But the demands of the coaches, parents, and the athletes themselves create a push toward perfection that contributes to the development of eating disorders, and the problem is clearly prevalent among these athletes.

Athletes in other sports have problems with eating disorders as well. William "Refrigerator" Perry, a defensive lineman with the Philadelphia Eagles, has struggled with compulsive overeating during his sports career. Runners, cyclists, swimmers, wrestlers, and others are at risk, too.

Often exercise addiction or the compulsion to exercise is part of the complex behavior of an eating disorder. An athlete may use exercise to purge himself or herself of calories instead of vomiting or using other means of controlling food intake.

WHY TEENS DEVELOP EATING DISORDERS

There are many reasons why a teen might develop an eating disorder. With a culture that is obsessed with appearance, it is hard not to become obsessed about your body and the way you look. Many teens develop eating disorders in an effort to improve their appearance through dieting. Dieting can quickly turn into an obsession with weight, counting calories, restricting food intake, or eating only certain kinds of foods. These are the behaviors that turn into an eating disorder.

Another reason that teens develop eating disorders is a need for control. At a time in your life when so many things seem beyond your control—the changes of puberty, the demands of family, the requirements of school—you look for something you can control. Although you are not aware of it at the time, dieting and focusing on what you can and cannot eat can be ways to control some areas of your life.

During the changes of puberty, there is little you can control about your body. You cannot control how tall you get, how much your nose grows, or how big your feet get. But to some extent you can control your weight. Teens also want to look good. You want to look like people you admire—role models such as celebrities and peers you think are cool. In many instances these role models are thin, as are many people you see in the movies, television shows, and magazines. Such people seem perfect. But look around you. People come in all different shapes and sizes.

EMOTIONAL AND PHYSICAL ABUSE

A teen may develop an eating disorder if he or she is in an abusive relationship or has been in one earlier in his or her life. The abuse may be physical, sexual, or emotional. Whatever the kind of abuse a person experiences, it has damaging effects on a person. The effects can last a long time and become hidden in the unconscious mind, so that the person is no longer aware of them. But the effects may surface in self-destructive or abusive behaviors, such as an eating disorder, exercise addiction, or chemical addiction. Abuse has a devastating effect on a person's self-esteem and self-image.

Abuse can be sexual. This includes inappropriate physical contact of any kind such as unwanted kissing, touching, or tickling, as well as inappropriate comments about your appearance, such as "you look sexy in that dress." Sexual abuse can include suggestive behavior that may not involve physical contact but feels inappropriate, such as adults walking around the house inappropriately dressed after a child is well into adolescence. Unusual restrictions on dating or peer contacts can be abusive.

Abuse may be physical, and it can include hitting, slapping, pushing, kicking, biting, or inflicting physical harm through the use of objects like belts and cigarettes. Even the mere threat of physical harm can be considered abuse. Emotional abuse includes name calling, berating, shaming or humiliating a person, or threatening a person. Berating a person includes any demeaning or negative comment that undermines a person's self-confidence, such as "you can't do anything right" or "you are always messing up." Telling a person to shut up all the time or telling a person that he or she is clumsy or incompetent is also abuse.

Abuse includes neglect, such as not tending to a person's physical, emotional, or intellectual needs.

Not showing an interest in a person's activities or friends, not encouraging a person to do well, or not setting appropriate limits like bedtimes and curfews are examples of neglect. Other examples include failing to get someone appropriate medical attention or not requiring that a child attend school.

Abuse affects your self-esteem and your self-image in profound ways. If someone is always telling you that you look overweight, you start to see yourself that way. Your self-image becomes one of an overweight person, no matter how much you weigh. Negative comments like this can lead to an eating disorder. When someone compliments or praises you, it makes you feel good about yourself. You learn to value yourself and are less likely to become involved in negative behaviors.

ANOREXIA NERVOSA

For many years some women and girls have been starving themselves to stay thin. But men as well as women can be anorexic. Approximately 90 to 95 percent of anorexia nervosa sufferers are girls and women. That means approximately 5 to 10 percent are boys and men.

Anorexia nervosa is the medical term for self-starvation as a way to control your weight. It is a complex problem that may include many behaviors about food and ways of thinking about food. Ritualistic eating is part of the pattern of anorexia nervosa. It includes eating only certain kinds of food, arranging your food on your plate in a certain way, cutting your food into tiny bits, and eating certain foods at certain times of the day.

Between 1 and 2 percent of American women suffer from anorexia nervosa at sometime during their lives. If left untreated, it is a serious disorder with life-threatening consequences. According to ANRED (Anorexia Nervosa and Related Eating Disorders), 20 percent of people with serious eating disorders die because they do not get treatment. The symptoms of anorexia nervosa include:

⊙ Refusal to maintain body weight at or above a normal weight

⊙ Intense fear of weight gain or being fat

⊙ Feeling fat or overweight despite dramatic weight loss

⊙ Loss of menstrual periods in postpuberty women and girls

⊙ Extreme concern with body weight and shape

WHAT HAPPENS WHEN A PERSON HAS ANOREXIA?

People with anorexia nervosa have a very distorted self-image. They continue to see themselves as overweight even as they are losing weight. They cannot look in a mirror and see themselves objectively. They tend to be perfectionists and are never thin enough, never perfect enough. Even as they lose pound after pound and their clothes hang loosely off their bony frames, they do not see how thin they are getting. They cannot stop their ritualistic eating and distorted thinking about food. Some researchers suggest that this is because of a chemical reaction that is occurring in the brain. Research is continuing in this area.

People with anorexia nervosa have a strange logic or way of thinking about food. Some refer to this as anorexic logic. For example, anorexics may think that they deserve to eat only certain kinds of food or that they will gain weight if they eat more than a certain number of calories, usually far below what is considered normal calorie intake.

Anorexic logic involves such behaviors as having only lettuce for dinner or allowing yourself only one slice of bread each week. The desire to eat alone is also common. Whatever the eating pattern of anorexics, they severely restrict the amount of food or calories that are taken in each day. Pains are taken to count the calories, often keeping careful records of all food intake. No matter how much weight anorexics lose, it is never enough. They still believe they have to lose more. They are not perfect.

Because a person with anorexia nervosa is not eating properly and not receiving proper nutrition, serious complications can develop. When the body is denied essential nutrients it needs for normal functioning, it slows down to conserve energy. Deprived of calories, it starts to feed on itself, depleting stores of fat. Eventually even the vital organs are affected. The health consequences of this process are severe and life-threatening. They include:

⊙ Abnormally slow heart rate and low blood pressure, which means that the heart muscle is changing. The risk for heart failure rises as the heart rate and blood pressure levels sink lower and lower.

⊙ Reduction of bone density (osteoporosis), which results in dry, brittle bones.

⊙ Muscle loss and weakness.

⊙ Severe dehydration, which can result in kidney failure.

⊙ Fainting, fatigue, and overall weakness.

⊙ Dry hair and skin; hair loss.

⊙ Growth of a downy layer of hair called lanugo all over the body, including the face, as the body tries to keep itself warm.

Anorexia nervosa is a serious problem. It has one of the highest death rates of any mental health condition. Between 5 and 20 percent of individuals struggling with anorexia nervosa will die. The probability of death increases within that range depending on how long the person has had the disorder.

CHECK YOURSELF

Here are the warning signs of anorexia nervosa:

⊙ Dramatic weight loss

⊙ Preoccupation with weight, food, calories, fat, and dieting

⊙ Refusal to eat certain foods, progressing to restrictions against whole categories of food (for example, no carbohydrates, fats, etc.)

⊙ Frequent comments about feeling overweight despite weight loss

⊙ Anxiety about gaining weight or being fat

⊙ Denial of hunger

⊙ Development of food rituals (such as eating foods in a certain order, excessive chewing, rearranging food on a plate)

⊙ Consistent excuses to avoid mealtimes or situations involving food

⊙ Avoidance of usual friends and withdrawal from activities

⊙ In general, behaviors and attitudes indicating that weight loss, dieting, and control of food are becoming primary concerns

⊙ Excessive, rigid exercise regimen, in spite of weather, fatigue, illness, or an injury

It may be hard to understand how people could let themselves get so thin that their bones stick out and their clothes hang loosely off their bodies. The person with anorexia nervosa has an illness. Even when the person seeks treatment, it is a difficult illness to treat. The person often has many setbacks and requires repeated hospitalizations. This is why early intervention is essential.

The sooner a person gets help for this disorder, the better his or her chances of recovery. If you think you might have a problem with an eating disorder, talk to your school nurse, counselor, physician, parent, or another responsible adult you feel comfortable talking to.

BULIMIA NERVOSA

Bulimia nervosa is a serious and potentially life-threatening eating disorder characterized by a cycle of bingeing and purging. Like anorexics, most bulimia sufferers are female. Approximately 80 percent of all those affected are female. Bulimia affects 1 to 3 percent of middle and high school girls and 1 to 4 percent of college-age women. About 20 percent of bulimics are males. More often, males suffer from a binge eating disorder or compulsive overeating that is not followed by purging.

Bulimia is a disorder that is easy to hide. People who have bulimia often appear to be of average body weight. They binge in secrecy and purge in a locked bathroom or purge by excessive exercising. Exercising is usually a healthy choice, and bulimics may even be encouraged and praised for working out. Bulimia nervosa has three primary symptoms:

⊙ Eating large quantities of food in short periods of time, often secretly, without regard to feelings of fullness or hunger, and to the point of feeling out of control while eating.

⊙ Binges are followed by some form of purging or compensatory behavior to make up for the excessive calories taken in. Purging can include self-induced vomiting, laxative or diuretic abuse, fasting, or compulsive exercise.

⊙ Extreme concern with body weight and shape.

People with bulimia nervosa often develop complex schedules or rituals to provide opportunities for binge and purge sessions. Unlike anorexics, bulimics often recognize that their behaviors are unusual and can be dangerous to their health.

HEALTH CONSEQUENCES OF BULIMIA NERVOSA

Because of the binge-purge nature of bulimia, over the long term this behavior can have serious effects on the body. Repeated gorging on food followed by abrupt purging through vomiting, laxatives, or diuretics is damaging to the entire digestive system. It damages the esophagus and teeth. It leads to electrolyte and chemical imbalances in the body that can affect the heart and other major organs. The health consequences of bulimia include:

⊙ Electrolyte imbalances that can lead to an irregular heartbeat and possibly heart failure and death. These imbalances are caused by losses of potassium and sodium from the body and dehydration as a result of purging behavior.

⊙ Inflammation and possible rupture of the esophagus from frequent vomiting.

⊙ Chronic irregular bowel movements and constipation as a result of laxative abuse.

⊙ Tooth decay and staining from stomach acids released during frequent vomiting.

⊙ Peptic ulcers and pancreatitis.

Bingeing and purging on food is more than a gimmick at sleepover parties or something you learn about when you go away to college. It is a serious problem that requires early intervention. Many people suffer from bulimia for years. They become obsessed with the need to purge themselves after eating. They cannot control the need to vomit, exercise, or use laxatives to rid themselves of food and calories.

CHECK YOURSELF

Here are the warning signs of bulimia nervosa:

⊙ Sneaking food from the kitchen or hiding food in a bedroom or school locker for a binge later

⊙ Eating large amounts of food in short periods of time, then hiding the existence of wrappers and containers

⊙ Runs to the bathroom after meals to purge, signs of vomiting, the presence of wrappers or packages of laxatives or diuretics

⊙ An excessive, rigid exercise regimen; exercising despite poor weather, fatigue, illness, and injury

⊙ Unusual swelling of the cheeks or jaw area

⊙ Calluses on the back of the hands and knuckles from self-induced vomiting

⊙ Discoloration of the teeth

⊙ Creation of complex lifestyle schedules or rituals to make time for binge-purge sessions

⊙ Withdrawal from friends and activities

⊙ Behaviors and attitudes indicating that weight loss, dieting, and control of food are becoming primary concerns

The chances for recovery increase with early detection of bulimia nervosa. Talk to a counselor, school nurse, physician, parent, or someone you can trust if you are suffering from this eating disorder.

EATING DISORDERS AND THE ELITE ATHLETE

The Olympics were a year off and Jonelee had one more year to train to get into top form. Competition was nothing new to Jonelee. She had been taking swimming classes since she was five years old. Her mom and dad called her their little Olympian. It was always her mother's dream to have an Olympic champion in the family. When Jonelee showed an interest in swimming after watching the summer Olympics, her mother rushed her to the nearest swim club to sign her up for classes.

Two years later they moved to Colorado so Jonelee could be closer to a world-class coach, the best in the country, many believed. Jonelee had to work hard to learn the new diving skills she needed. She wasn't a "natural" like some in her class for whom the twists and somersaults came easily. But she was determined to do well. She worked hard and demanded the most of herself. She was going to make it to the Olympics someday and make her parents proud of her.

The new coach was as tough as people said. He demanded the best of his divers. But Jonelee worked hard. By the time she was fourteen she was one of the best in her diving class. Coach Miller said she had good things ahead of her if she trained hard and didn't slack off. She might make the next Olympic team.

Coach Miller had nicknames for everyone to get them to work harder. Jonelee had a good appetite and Coach Miller jokingly called her "little Miss Piggy." Soon he added things like "You've got a little roll under your chin, Miss Piggy, and you'll never make it off the end of the board" or "What did you have for dinner last night, your meatballs and your brother's, too?" It stung when he said things like that and Jonelee had to push back the tears. But she figured he was just trying to help her do her best. He joked with everybody about their weight.

When puberty hit, Jonelee had to work even harder to keep her weight down. As she grew, she gained muscle weight and bone mass. To compensate, Jonelee went on a strict diet. At first it was easy. Jonelee skipped a few meals and quickly lost three pounds, thanks to her vigorous training schedule. Then it got more difficult. She started to skip lunch. Then it was a slice of bread with cheese for dinner. She added diuretics to lose water weight, especially during her period, and took diet pills to control her appetite. Soon Jonelee could not eat a meal without becoming guilt-ridden and terrified about gaining weight. She became obsessed with her weight and was locked into a cycle of fasting and diet pills.

In college Jane Fonda started taking Dexedrine, then called a "pep pill" but today known as speed, which decreased her appetite and gave her energy. While modeling, Fonda learned about diuretics, and she continued to take them for twenty years. She developed a tolerance for them and had to take more to achieve the same effect.

EXERCISE AS A PURGING BEHAVIOR

Many teens with eating disorders use exercise to purge themselves of calories instead of vomiting. Others use exercise to lose weight as a symptom of the eating disorder anorexia nervosa. Compulsive exercise must be treated along with the eating disorder. A teen who stops compulsively exercising will likely start purging in other ways unless the eating disorder is treated.

9 Treating Exercise Addiction

Think back to when you first started exercising. Once you began a regular workout routine, you liked the way it made you feel. You liked working out until you sweat. It made you feel kind of high, invigorated, and clear-headed.

The physical benefits made it that much better. Toned muscles and fresh looking skin made you look great and you burned off calories in the process. Working out was great. You couldn't get enough of it. It had other payoffs, too, like boosting your self-confidence and making you feel good about yourself. You even decided to try out for a sports team at school. Working out was so appealing, you got hooked on it. Then everything you did had to be planned around your workout schedule. You couldn't do anything until you planned your next thirty-minute run. Exercise had become the number one activity in your life. Suddenly you felt out of control, compelled to exercise even though you no longer enjoyed it.

TREATING EXERCISE ADDICTION

Exercise addiction has many similarities to other addictions. Each of these addictive behaviors involves an obsessive preoccupation with satisfying a craving and the neglect of family, friends, social responsibilities, work, and school. Addictive behaviors usually involve physical risks as well.

A person addicted to exercise is preoccupied with his or her exercise workout. The exercise addict usually focuses exclusively on one sport or exercise routine. He or she spends a lot of time thinking about exercising and schedules all of his or her activities around the next workout. The person addicted to exercise neglects social relationships, school, and work to pursue his or her craving for exercise. The physical consequences of overexercising include repeated injuries, fatigue and exhaustion, degeneration of muscles, and long-term hip and joint injuries.

The person who is addicted to exercise denies that a problem exists. "How can you be addicted to exercise, something that is good for you?" The person with an exercise addiction tends to avoid treatment for the compulsion but sees a physician for the treatment of injuries so that he or she can get back to a regular exercise routine. Dr. Rick Aberman says that people come to see him because of injuries when they are not able to exercise. They are experiencing depression, anxiety, and irritability—in other words, withdrawal symptoms.

EXERCISE AND TEEN DEVELOPMENT

If you tell exercise addicts to quit running, they will never come back, says Dr. Aberman. According to

Aberman, success in treating exercise addiction means understanding that the runner, the cyclist, the dancer, the golfer, the tennis player, or the weight lifter wants to be able to continue his or her activities. Even if people no longer enjoy their workouts, they want to be able to recapture the feeling of pleasure they had from exercising when they started working out.

To treat the person with an exercise addiction, you have to look at why that person is exercising. The motivations behind the addiction are usually related to teen development problems, says Aberman. Developmental issues for teens include a growing need to be socially involved with peers. You are growing away from your parents and becoming more independent. You are developing your individuality and unique qualities by pursuing your interests, talents, and special skills. The onset of puberty and its many physical and emotional changes is a significant developmental issue for teens. Developmental issues are affected by what is going on in your family. If you are experiencing a lot of stress at home, you may be exercising to get away from these stresses.

Transitional times have an impact on developmental issues, too. Going from middle school to junior high or to high school is a major transition. So is the much anticipated graduation from high school. A teen athlete who has had a lot of success competing at the high school level but who finds himself not good enough to compete at the college level could become obsessed with exercise in an effort to overcome his disadvantage.

One approach to treating exercise addiction is

to address the developmental issues first. These developmental issues may have triggered the exercise addiction. A teen who is experiencing problems at home, for example, may focus all of his or her pent-up anger and frustration into a sport or exercise workout.

Another approach to treating exercise addiction is to break down the addict's belief in the goal of a perfect body by teaching a new attitude toward working out. The goal of working out becomes one of nurturing the body, not making it perfect. If you exercise with the belief "no pain, no gain," you have to change that goal. You don't have to work out until you are in pain, sore, or overworked to get the full benefit of a workout. Instead, use your workouts to increase your body awareness. How does your body feel as you exercise? Did you stretch enough before you started? Can you feel your muscles warming up, getting stronger? Use your workout time to get in touch with your feelings. Did you feel stressed when you started to exercise? Can you feel yourself relaxing as you move and enjoy the workout? If you were angry when you started, can you feel yourself letting go of the anger as you get into the stride of your run? Try to enjoy the physical sensations of working out. The goal is to go from "I have to exercise" to "I want to exercise, and I have a choice."

When you have problems with your self-image, you can shift the focus of your exercise from working to have a perfect body to enjoying your body and the pleasure of working out. As you work out, try to enjoy the feeling and process of moving your body, rather than exercising to burn

calories and escape from your feelings of imper-
fection. You also have to create a realistic picture
in your head of what a healthy body looks like.
You have to accept that a certain amount of body
fat is necessary for a healthy body.

Put pictures up on the walls of your room and in
your school locker of people with regular bodies, not
models with the kind of perfect bodies that most
people don't have the money or time to achieve.

Karin Kratina, an exercise physiologist in
Coconut Creek, Florida, suggests that you try to
look at what you are really feeling—hurt, anger, or
sadness—and process the feelings and work on the
problems that are causing those feelings. As you
heal, give yourself time to adjust to a new way of
exercising. Remind yourself that healing is an
ongoing process. Like other addictions, the old
triggers—the events that created the urge to work
out excessively—will continue to make you want to
exercise. If you learn what makes you want to exercise excessively—what your triggers are—you will
learn new ways to react instead.

THE TREATMENT PLAN

When you change your exercise goals, you change
the focus of your addiction. Instead of being
obsessed about your body and your appearance,
you can learn to exercise for health and enjoyment. Look at the issues that are contributing to
your exercise addiction. Are you exercising to
avoid problems at home? Do you exercise
because you do not have any friends and do not
know how to make new ones? Are you exercising

because you like the competitive goals that you set for yourself? Are you obsessed with your appearance and trying to exercise your way to a perfect body? If you do not know why you exercise, try this experiment. If you spontaneously exercise in response to events that are occurring, you may be exercising to deal with stress. Did you just eat a big piece of cake? You may be exercising to burn calories or to purge.

CHECK YOURSELF

Keep a log of what happens immediately before and after you exercise. Jot down what you are doing before you exercise. What event preceded your desire to exercise? Did you just have a fight with your parents? Did you flunk a test at school and immediately come home and grab your tennis racket? Record what you are feeling. Are you angry, sad, disappointed, scared? Immediately after you exercise, record the next event. Then record what you are feeling.

Recording your thoughts during this time can help you to understand how you use exercise. Looking at the events before and after you exercise and how you feel about them can help you understand what issues you are dealing with by over-exercising. Making changes in your workout routine can help you successfully return to an exercise program that is manageable and healthy. While working on these changes, be sure to allow yourself time to make adjustments to your workout routine. It is best to change one area of your workout at a time.

Change Your Exercise Goals

Instead of exercising to sculpt the perfect body, make your exercise a time for recreation and enjoyment.

- ⊙ Put the focus of exercising back on enjoyment and physical health.

- ⊙ Channel your need for perfection into other areas like hobbies or school.

- ⊙ Slowly stop keeping records of your workouts.

- ⊙ Do not track miles or distances. Run for forty-five minutes, not five miles. Keep the focus on how long you are going to run and relax, not on how far you are going to run or how many laps you will swim.

- ⊙ Look around you as you work out, enjoy the scenery and the way your body moves. Make working out a plea- surable experience.

- ⊙ Make your workout a social event. Talk to the person you walk past on the walking trail. Say hello to the guy who is swimming in the lap lane next to you.

- ⊙ Take the focus of your workout off self- improvement and concentrate on your enjoyment of physical activity.

Change the Times of Your Exercise Schedule

Changing the times of your workout routine is important. You need to become flexible about working out if you want to overcome compulsive exercising.

⊙ Change the days of your workouts. Keep changing the days and continue to do so. Try to get flexible in your scheduling.

⊙ Change the length of time that you have scheduled for exercise once in a while, but not every time you work out. Keep focused on exercising for recreation and health, not on psychological need to exercise a set amount of time.

⊙ Schedule some other activity for the time when you would have been exercising. Go to the library. Walk your dog. Work on your homework. Plan something else to do.

⊙ Coping with unstructured time is difficult for the exercise addict, but you must teach yourself to do it.

Change the Kind of Exercising You Do

You can continue to use some of your exercise time for the sport or activity that you love, but try to add other activities as well. In other words, cross-train. Every other day add walking to your workout activities instead of cycling. Get involved in coaching a team or volunteering to help at sporting events, rather than concentrating exclusively on personal physical activity.

Use Other Means to Reduce Stress

Learn what causes you to feel stress and learn other ways to manage your stress. Learn to identify your stress triggers. What makes you feel stress? Check your body reactions to learn when you are feeling stress and identify what event is occurring or has occurred to cause the stress. Use stress management techniques. Look at the way you talk about yourself. Do you have a lot of negative thoughts? Change the negative ones into positive ones. Practice deep breathing and muscle relaxation. Get therapy or join a support group if your anxiety and depression are unmanageable.

Schedule Exercise

Though you may have varied your exercise routine to break up obsessive patterns, sometimes the opposite strategy helps. If you are spontaneously running to the track or the pool every time something puts you in a bad mood, you may need to build a regular structure into your exercise routine to avoid surrendering to these cravings for exercise on a moment's notice.

Try scheduling your workouts at regular times. Don't react to anxiety or depression by putting on your running shoes. Instead, try to look at problems that may be contributing to your moods and try new strategies for dealing with them. If you exercise to purge and burn calories, set regular exercise times so that you cannot impulsively exercise after a binge.

Get Help

Problems with ongoing depression, anxiety, or eating disorders will continue to show up in some way even if you are managing your exercise addiction well. You could easily become cross-addicted to some other activity or some other form of compulsive behavior. Therapy options include individual therapy, group therapy, behavioral therapy, medications, or support groups like Overeaters Anonymous.

Change Your Body Image

Exercising for perfection is an unachievable goal. Try to look at your body realistically and practice accepting it.

- ☉ Look at your thoughts and the things you say about yourself and your body. For every negative thought about yourself, add a positive one. Follow "I have fat thighs" with "My legs are strong and I like how long they are."

- ☉ Separate your feelings about your body from your self-worth, your happiness, and your future success. No matter how fit you are, it will not make you happy for long or make you successful or increase your self-worth.

- ☉ Try to set a realistic image of your body, to see yourself as you really are, and to accept that. Look around you. People come in all different sizes and shapes and none of them are perfect.

⊙ Learn what your normal body weight should be and accept that 25 percent body fat is normal and healthy. Healthy and model-perfect are not the same thing.

⊙ Stop wearing shapeless clothes and practice wearing things that show off your body and that make you feel good because of their color or style.

Eat Three Meals a Day

Establishing regular meal times is a step toward managing eating disorders and compulsive exercising.

⊙ Eat three meals a day and a snack in between meals. In the beginning, you can allow yourself to have fewer calories as you adjust to this new schedule.

⊙ Gradually add calories to your meals.

⊙ Write down the times when you eat meals, but don't count calories. Try not to go more than three hours between eating meals or having a snack.

10

A Balanced Lifestyle

Exercise addiction presents a unique challenge to the sports enthusiast. You want to be able to exercise, yet you tend to overdo it. You tend to exercise compulsively, to the point of exhaustion or injury or both. But with treatment for exercise addiction, you have taken control over your workout routine and you are now exercising for recreation and enjoyment. Now you want to continue to workout without the risk of overdoing it, of becoming addicted again.

The keys to a manageable work out program are having a balanced lifestyle that includes many activities. When you change the goal of your exercise workouts, you have time to develop your other interests. Having a balanced lifestyle means that you participate in a variety of activities that meet your different needs.

As a teen there are many developmental issues that you are working on. You are becoming more independent and making your way in the world. Although you need the comfort and security of your family, you want to spend more time with your friends and peers. Your social needs are focused on dating, sleep-overs, and parties. You are also developing your skills and special talents. Your need to learn and excel is focused on school, after school activities, and work.

You want to stretch your body, learn new skills, and participate in physical activities. You hope to make the pep squad or basketball team to be with your friends and enjoy sports. You need a connection to a church, synagogue, or some other institution to develop your spiritual needs. You need connections to your community. When you are addicted to exercising, your focus is on exercise and working out. Now you have time to develop these other areas of your life, to satisfy your social needs, develop talents and skills, and make connections to others.

MAKING NEW SOCIAL CONTACTS

If you have been focusing your exercise workout on a sport that does not involve interaction with others, change to team sports and other activities. Change your workout at least two to three days a week to include activities where you interact with others. Instead of cycling the trail by yourself, join a bike club. Schedule bike rides with friends and try new bike trails and routes. Ride your bike for the time spent with friends, not to rack up a certain number of miles every day.

For running, try participating in events where you meet people and socialize during the event. Add hiking and walking nature trails to your workout activities and look for group activities that include these kinds of events.

Instead of participating in a sporting activity, coach a youth sports team or assist at a sporting event. Instead of running in the next 5K run, volunteer to hand out drinks at a rest station along the race route. Instead of lifting weights every day, agree to help coach other kids who are learning to use the weight machines. Volunteer to help keep score and run the time clock at the basketball tournament. Contact the parks and recreation department in your area to see if there are other ways you can become involved in sporting activities. Organize a softball team with your friends. Put the focus of your interest in sports and working out into other sports activities.

SCHOOL AND WORK ACTIVITIES

Devote some of the energy you have been putting into working out into improving your school work or finding a part-time job. Change your routine and workout schedule. If you usually lift weights every day after school, get a part-time job at least three days a week.

Get involved in school organizations. Have you always wanted to try acting but never had the time to be in a play because of your workout schedule? Talk to the drama teacher and find out about auditions for the next school play. If you don't want to be on stage, ask if you can help work on the set or props for the show. Join the chess club, take a speech or debate class, help your friend win a student election, or run for class office yourself.

TALENTS AND SPECIAL SKILLS

Have you always wanted to take guitar lessons but never had the time? As you change your schedule and focus from exercise to new activities, you will be free to take guitar lessons. Maybe what you really want to do is start a band. If you take guitar lessons or other lessons that will develop your musical skills, you can start a band or join one that you like. Do you love science? Join the science club. Do you like working at your computer? You can develop an interest in computers by taking a class about writing computer programs, developing software, or creating a Web site. Do you like to work on cars? Try taking an auto mechanics class and turn the interest into a part-time job. Do you love horses? Look for a part-time job on a ranch or farm. Take riding lessons.

GETTING INVOLVED IN YOUR RELIGION AND COMMUNITY

If your parents have been encouraging you to get more involved in your church or synagogue, there are many ways you can do so. Instead of focusing exclusively on your exercise program, you can spend time on spiritual activities. Most houses of worship have youth groups that you can join. If you like to sing, you could join the choir. Check out what volunteer work the church or synagogue is doing and see if you can participate. Baby-sit in the nursery during services and activities.

Getting involved in your community is a great way to add new activities to your schedule. The parks and recreation department has many activities and programs you can get involved in. If your community does not have a parks and recreation department, it may have a summer Little League program or a youth soccer league. Check out the opportunities that are available to become involved in sports programs in your community.

Many organizations and community groups include activities for young people. If there is a boys or girls club in your area, they welcome volunteers. Other groups like Meals on Wheels use volunteers to bring meals to the homebound. Habitat for Humanity is run mostly by volunteers who build homes for people in need. The local community center, hospital, nursing home, or homeless shelter also welcomes volunteers. The library may have volunteer opportunities. During the school year you could read to children during story hour. Learn about the summer reading program at the library and volunteer to participate. If there is no program like this in your area, you could start one.

There may be a branch of 4-H in your area. They have many activities and events to participate in. You could volunteer to work with a younger brother's or sister's Boy Scout or Girl Scout troop. Civic or business organizations may have programs for young people. Political groups, citizen action groups, and environmental groups are another way to get involved in the community.

A HEALTHY EXERCISE PROGRAM

Part of having a balanced and healthy life is having an appropriate exercise program. Now that your exercise addiction is manageable, you want to continue to enjoy your sporting activities. According to Dr. J. Morrow and Dr. Philip Harvey, clinical psychologists who specialize in sports psychology, compulsive exercisers should focus on five ideas to change the way they look at exercise:

1. There is a need for rest days in any good fitness program.

2. Choosing to rest gives you more, not less, control over your life.

3. A certain amount of body fat is healthy and aesthetically appealing.

4. Success and happiness in life usually have little to do with a person's body condition or level of fitness.

5. Beyond a certain point, increasing exercise will not significantly increase its benefits.

Keeping a healthy exercise routine means keeping your focus on exercise as a form of recreation and entertainment, not as a way to change your body image or achieve perfection.

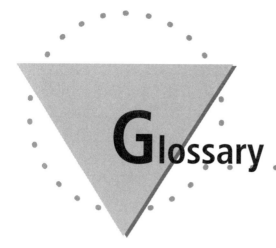

Glossary

aerobic activity   Any activity that raises the heart rate and increases breathing and supplies oxygen to the body for an extended period of time, usually twenty or more minutes.

anorexia nervosa   A type of disordered eating where a person severely limits his or her intake of calories out of an intense fear of gaining weight.

binge   To overindulge in an activity, often associated with food.

bulimia nervosa   A type of disordered eating where a person engages in a cycle of bingeing on food and then purging himself or herself of the food intake. Purging commonly involves vomiting, diuretics, laxatives, or exercise.

cardiovascular   Having to do with the heart and the fitness of the heart.

compulsive behavior   A behavior or activity that a person needs to repeat over and over again.

Compulsive behavior can lead to an addiction to a substance or activity.

compulsive exercise   A physical activity or exercise that a person needs to repeat over and over again. Not engaging in the physical activity creates anxiety in the individual and results in withdrawal symptoms.

cross-training   Participating in several sports activities and exercises as part of an overall fitness plan to develop total body fitness.

denial   A common defense mechanism for addiction where a person denies that he or she has a problem. Usually the person does not believe that he or she does have a problem until confronted with the consequences of his or her addictive behavior.

physical fitness   A certain level of physical development and training that allows one to engage in various physical activities with a minimum of difficulty.

puberty   From the Latin pubes, which means adult; the physical and emotional changes a person goes through during adolescence in the process of becoming an adult.

purge   Behavior that is part of an eating disorder where a person rids himself or herself of food or calories. Purging usually involves self-induced vomiting, diuretics or laxatives, or excessive exercising.

ritualistic eating   Eating behavior that is part of an eating disorder. It includes the compulsive need to restrict the kinds of food one eats; how one eats food, such as cutting food into tiny pieces; and when and where one eats food.

tolerance   An aspect of addictive behavior in which the need for an activity or substance increases because the body has become used to that substance or activity and feels its effect less and less.

withdrawal   The physical and emotional reactions to not engaging in an addictive behavior or taking an addictive substance.

Where to Go for Help

American Anorexia/Bulimia Association
165 W. 46th Street, Suite 1108
New York, NY 10036
(212) 575-6200

American College of Sports Medicine
P.O. Box 1440
Indianapolis, IN 46206-1440
(317) 637-9200

American Running and Fitness Association
4405 East West Highway, Suite 405
Bethesda, MD 20814

Anorexia Nervosa and Related Eating
    Disorders (ANRED)
P.O. Box 5102
Eugene, OR 97405
(503) 344-1144

Bulimia and Anorexia Self Help (BASH)
6125 Clayton Avenue
Suite 215
St. Louis, MO 63139
(314) 567-4080

Center for the Study of Anorexia and Bulimia
1 W. 91st Street
New York, NY 10024
(212) 595-3449

Eating Disorders Awareness and Prevention, Inc.
603 Steward Street
Suite 803
Seattle, WA 98101
(206) 382-3587

Foundation for Education About Eating Disorders
    (FEED)
P.O. Box 16375
Baltimore, MD 21210
(410) 467-0603

National Association of Anorexia Nervosa and
    Associated Disorders (ANAD)
P.O. Box 7
Highland Park, IL 00035

The Renfrew Center
(800) REN-FREW
Residential, partial, and outpatient programs in
Philadelphia, New York City, Long Island, New Jersey,
and Florida

Newsgroups
alt.recovery.compulsive-eat
alt.support.big-folks
alt.support.eating-disord

Eating Disorders Listserve
e-mail to listserv@netcom
message "subscribe eatdis-1"

For Further Reading

Books

Baer, Judy. *Fill My Empty Heart.* Minneapolis: Bethany House Publishers, 1990.

Berg, Frances M. *Afraid to Eat: Children and Teens in Weight Crisis.* Hettinger, ND: Healthy Weight Journal, 1997.

Bode, Janet. *Food Fight.* New York: Simon & Schuster, 1997.

Cooke, Kaz. *Real Gorgeous: The Truth About Body & Beauty.* New York: W.W. Norton & Company, 1996.

Fonda, Jane. *Jane Fonda's Workout Book.* New York: Simon & Schuster, 1981.

Hirschmann, Jar R., and Carol H. Munter. *When Women Stop Hating Their Bodies.* New York: Fawcett Columbine, 1995.

Kaminker, Laura. *Exercise Addiction: When Fitness Becomes an Obsession.* New York: Rosen Publishing Group, 1998.

LeMieux, Anne C. *Dare to Be M.E.* New York: Avon Books, 1997.

Maloney, Michael, M.D., and Rachel Kranz. *Straight Talk About Eating Disorders.* New York: Dell Publishing, 1991.

Moe, Barbara. *Coping with Eating Disorders.* New York: Rosen Publishing Group, 1999.

Prussing, Rebecca, Philip Harvey, et al. *Hooked on Exercise.* New York: Simon & Schuster, 1992.

131

Ryan, Joan. *Little Girls in Pretty Boxes: The Making and Breaking of Elite Gymnasts and Figure Skaters.* New York: Doubleday, 1995.

Valette, Brett. *A Parent's Guide to Eating Disorders.* New York: Walker Publishing Co., 1988.

Magazine Articles

Anderson, Judith. "Why Aren't Eating Disorders a National Health Priority?" *Glamour,* Vol. 92, Issue 3, March 1994, p. 139.

Applegate, Liz, "Running Into Trouble." *Runner's World,* Vol. 33, Issue 4, April 1998, pp. 30-33.

Bell, Alison. "Eating Disorders and the Toll They're Taking on Teens." *Teen,* February 1999, pp. 65-71.

Brown-Goebeler, S. "Pursuit of Perfection." *Time,* Vol. 30, November 18, 1991, pp. 88-90.

Grant, Elenor. "The Exercise Fix." *Psychology Today,* February 1988, pp. 24-28.

Iknoian, Therese. "What Ails Women Athletes?" *American Health,* Vol. 12, Issue 8, October 1993, p. 55.

Israel, Betsy. "Two Girls Talk About Food, Fat, Bodies, and 'Bones.'" *Redbook,* Vol. 189, Issue 6, October 1997, pp. 123-124.

Morrow, J., Ph.D., and Philip Harvey, Ph.D. "Hooked on Exercise, Part II." *American Health,* July/August 1991.

Peterson, Karen S. "Knowledgeable Teens Still Starve for Attention." *USA Today,* July 18, 1997, pp. 8D.

Philpott, David, and Glenn Sheppard. "More Than Mere Vanity: Men with Eating Disorders." *Guidance & Counseling,* Vol. 13, Issue 4, Summer 1998, pp. 28-34.

Rotwien, Randi E. "Obsessed with Exercise." *Idea Today,* Vol. 13, Issue 8, September 1995, pp. 57-60.

Schien, Pamela with Jeff Copeland. "I Am an Exercise Addict." *Fitness,* March/April 1994, pp. 66-69.

Stark, Elizabeth. "Working It Out." *Mademoiselle,* January 1993.

Index

133